Community emergency preparedness: a manual for managers and policy-makers

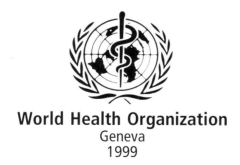

World Health Organization
Geneva
1999

WHO Library Cataloguing-in-Publication Data

Community emergency preparedness : a manual for managers and policy-makers.
1.Emergencies 2.Emergency medical services – organization and administration 3.Policy making 4.Consumer participation 5.Administrative personnel 6.Manuals

ISBN 92 4 154519 4 (NLM Classification: WB 105)

The World Health Organization welcomes requests for permission to reproduce or translate its publications, in part or in full. Applications and enquiries should be addressed to the Office of Publications, World Health Organization, Geneva, Switzerland, which will be glad to provide the latest information on any changes made to the text, plans for new editions and reprints and translations already available.

© **World Health Organization 1999**

Publications of the World Health Organization enjoy copyright protection in accordance with the provisions of Protocol 2 of the Universal Copyright Convention. All rights reserved.

The designations employed and the presentation of the material in this publication do not imply the expression of any opinion whatsoever on the part of the Secretariat of the World Health Organization concerning the legal status of any country, territory, city or area or of its authorities, or concerning the delimitation of its frontiers or boundaries.

The mention of specific companies or of certain manufacturers' products does not imply that they are endorsed or recommended by the World Health Organization in preference to others of a similar nature that are not mentioned. Errors and omissions excepted, the names of proprietary products are distinguished by initial capital letters.

Typeset in Hong Kong
Printed in Malta
97/11785 – Best-set/Interprint – 7500

Contents

Preface	v
Acknowledgements	vi

Chapter 1
Introduction

Decision-making for emergency preparedness	1
What is emergency preparedness?	12
Community participation	15
Project management	17
Summary	18
References	19

Chapter 2
Policy development

Policy	20
Emergency preparedness policy	20
Issues in emergency management policy	21
Summary	28
Reference	29

Chapter 3
Vulnerability assessment

Introduction	30
The process of vulnerability assessment	32
The planning group	34
Hazard identification	38
Hazard description	39
Describing the community	54
Description of effects and vulnerability	57
Hazard prioritization	60
Recommending action	67
Summary	68
References	68

Chapter 4
Emergency planning

Introduction	70
An emergency planning process	73
Planning group review	75
Potential problem analysis	75
Resource analysis	78
Roles and responsibilities	79
Management structure	81
Strategies and systems	83
Content of community emergency plans	104
Summary	106
References	106

Chapter 5
Training and education

Introduction	108
A systematic approach to training	108
Public education	111
Summary	111
References	112

Chapter 6
Monitoring and evaluation

Introduction	113
Project management	113
Checklists	115
Exercises	115
Summary	117

Annexes

1. Project management	118
2. Hazard description tables	121
3. Emergency preparedness checklists	130
4. Personal protection in different types of emergencies	138

Preface

This manual is designed to assist those concerned with preparing for emergencies at the local level. It explains what emergency preparedness is and how to achieve it in an effective, appropriate way. It is intended principally for:

— local organizations and managers responsible for emergency planning (e.g. health sector administrators, directors of public works organizations, hospital administrators, and heads of volunteer organizations); and
— national and international officials involved in emergency management.

National civil protection bodies, emergency management organizations, and sectoral departments, such as public health authorities, are responsible for ensuring the safety and security of a nation's people, resources, and environment in the face of hazards. It is at the community level, however, that the full effects of emergencies are felt, and it is there that definitive achievements in emergency preparedness can be made. It is difficult for national and international emergency organizations to form an effective working relationship with a community that is unaware of its hazards and unprepared for emergencies.

The key to emergency preparedness is the involvement and commitment of all relevant individuals and organizations at every level — community, provincial, national, and international. This multisectoral approach means that many organizations accept clearly-defined responsibilities and the need to coordinate their efforts. Without their involvement and commitment, emergency preparedness becomes fragmented, inefficient, and poorly coordinated.

Self-evidently, one of the principal effects of any emergency will be on the health of the population. Preparedness within the health sector was felt to be beyond the scope of this manual; a separate WHO publication devoted entirely to health sector preparedness is planned.

The term "emergency" in this manual is used in the broadest possible sense. One person's emergency may be another's mere incident, and disasters cause problems above and beyond smaller emergencies. Nevertheless, the processes of emergency preparedness can be used to develop systems and programmes for coping with every scale of adverse events. Similarly, the same preparedness processes can be used for enhancing the safety of a building, a community, or an entire country.

This manual explains the processes of policy development, vulnerability assessment, emergency planning, training and education, and monitoring and evaluation for use in a wide range of emergency management applications.

Acknowledgements

This manual is the result of a lengthy process of research, consultation, and writing. WHO collaborated with a number of organizations during this process, including the International Civil Defense Organisation and the International Federation of Red Cross and Red Crescent Societies. Several experts contributed to elaborating the concepts included in the text and many others reviewed it and helped finalize its content. Dr S. Ben Yahmed, formerly Chief of Emergency Preparedness at WHO, developed the idea for the manual and coordinated the effort, which greatly benefited from the contributions and advice of Dr R. Doran (formerly, Division of Emergency and Humanitarian Action, WHO) and Professor E. Quarantelli (University of Delaware).

Contributions were also made by WHO's regional offices and by the WHO divisions responsible for such areas as operational support in environmental health, nutrition, communicable diseases, and mental health.

Special acknowledgement is due to: Mr M. Tarrant (Australian Emergency Management Institute) and Mr B. Dutton (Disaster Management Consultants International) for managing the development of the hazard analysis process that formed the basis of Chapter 3, Vulnerability assessment; the Disaster Management Consultants International team for technical editing; Mr J. Lunn, Mr B. Dutton, Mr W.A. Dodds, and Mr G. Marsh for developing the planning process that formed the basis of Chapter 4, Emergency planning; and Mr P. Koob (Disaster Management Consultants International) for writing the manual.

Chapter 1
Introduction

Decision-making for emergency preparedness
The increase in global vulnerability

Major emergencies and disasters have occurred throughout history and, as the world's population grows and resources become more limited, communities are increasingly vulnerable to the hazards that cause disasters. Statistics gathered since 1969 show a rise in the number of people affected by disasters (see Fig. 1). However, since there is little evidence that the actual events causing disasters are increasing in either intensity or frequency, it can only be concluded that vulnerability to disasters is growing.

Emergencies and disasters do not affect only health and well-being; frequently, large numbers of people are displaced, killed or injured, or subjected to greater risk of epidemics. Considerable economic harm is also common, and Fig. 2 shows how economic and insured losses have risen since 1960. This has led to a restructuring of the insurance industry, with insured parties bearing more costs, and governments assisting the insurance and reinsurance markets (2). Uninsured and economic losses are creating immense burdens on communities, economies, and governments. As Fig. 3 shows, these disasters are not confined to a particular part of the world; they can occur anywhere and at any time.

A disaster can be defined as any occurrence that causes damage, ecological disruption, loss of human life or deterioration of health and health services on a scale sufficient to warrant an extraordinary response from outside the affected community or area (3).

A recent Latin American study indicated that for each disaster listed in officially recognized disaster databases, there are some 20 other smaller emergencies with destructive impact on local communities that are unacknowledged. Hence, the actual harm caused by emergencies and disasters probably far outweighs the accepted disaster statistics.[1]

Disasters are causing greater harm to people, communities, and countries every decade, affecting current populations and existing infrastructure and threatening the future of sustainable development.

Clearly, neither communities nor governments can afford to wait for emergencies and disasters to occur before responding to them. The suffering caused by injuries

---
[1] Maskrey A. Communication at Seventh Scientific and Technical Meeting of the International Decade for Natural Disaster Reduction, Paris, 1995.

Fig. 1. **Number of people reported annually as affected by disasters**[a]

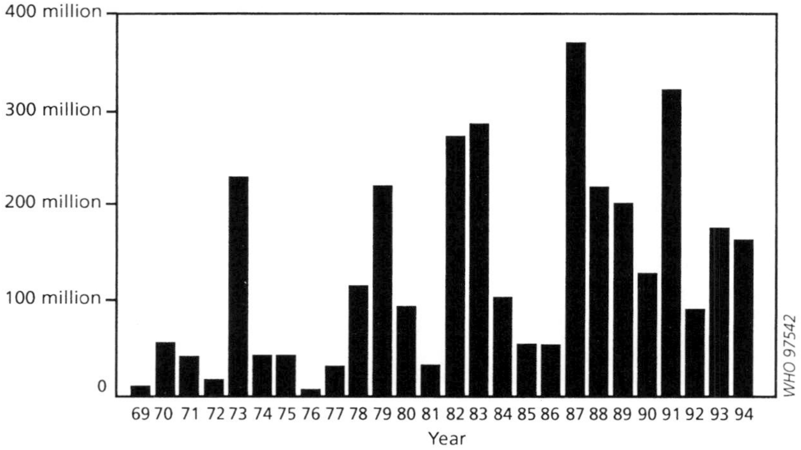

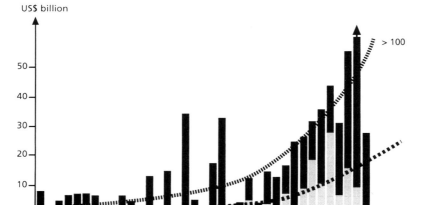

[a] Reproduced from reference 1 by permission of the publisher.

Fig. 2. **Economic and insured losses from natural disasters, 1960–1996**[a]

■ Economic losses (1996 values)
⋯⋯ Trend
▫ Insured losses (1996 values)
▪▪▪▪ Trend

[a] Reproduced from reference 2 by permission of the publisher.

Fig. 3. **Number of disasters with natural and non-natural triggers by global region in 1994**[a]

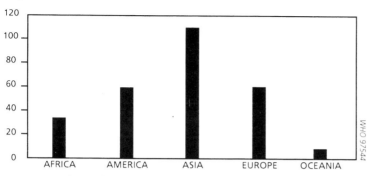

[a] Reproduced from reference 1 by permission of the publisher.

Fig. 4. **Value of humanitarian assistance (in US$) by year**[a]

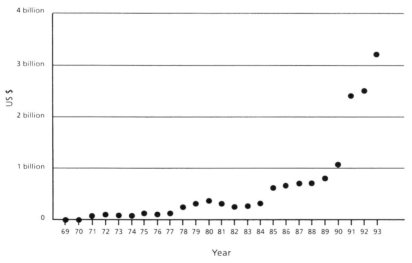

[a] Reproduced from reference 1 by permission of the publisher.

and deaths, social and economic disruption, and the destruction of the environment can be reduced through various measures designed to reduce vulnerability.

The effects of inappropriate humanitarian assistance

Often, the international community's reaction to disasters is to provide large amounts of humanitarian assistance and increased aid to the affected countries or communities. This might appear a fairly simple solution — to reduce short-term suffering and allow the community to rebuild. Figure 4 shows how humanitarian assistance has increased over the last three decades, from US$ 3 million in 1969 to US$ 3.2 billion in 1993. In 1995, it exceeded US$ 4 billion. Estimates show that, in 1980, global humanitarian assistance formed less than 1% of total overseas development assistance and that this figure had increased to 7% in 1993 (4).

Fig. 5. **How humanitarian assistance can increase vulnerability**

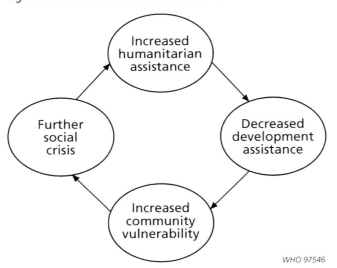

Frequently, humanitarian assistance takes the following course. It is not requested by the affected country and not integrated with the country's normal services or with community development. Assistance funds are diverted from those otherwise provided for development, thus reducing development opportunities in areas most vulnerable to emergencies and disasters. Delivery channels that parallel existing national channels are established for allocating and managing these assistance funds, leading to inefficiency and undermining existing development programmes. Hence, humanitarian assistance that is not properly coordinated at the national and community level can increase vulnerability and lead to greater dependence on further assistance, further social crises — and a need for *more* humanitarian assistance (see Fig. 5).

Badly coordinated humanitarian assistance clearly is not the answer and is a poor investment of time, resources, and money. Effective emergency preparedness, however, built in at an early stage, can establish the necessary structures and processes for an affected country to integrate humanitarian aid — provided *only* when requested — within its infrastructure in a cost-effective manner.

Vulnerability reduction and the focus on communities at risk

Coordinated efforts are also needed to halt emergencies and disasters by tackling the source — the deteriorating environment, the hazards that bring harm to communities, the vulnerability of communities to those hazards. Such efforts may be collectively termed "vulnerability reduction".

Vulnerability concerns the interaction between a community, its environment, and hazards. A community is the smallest social grouping in a country with an effective social structure and potential administrative capacity. The environment is the surrounding support system and processes. Hazards are the potential sources of emergencies of natural, technological, or social origin. A community

INTRODUCTION

interacts with its environment and its hazards. This interaction can be positive, resulting in vulnerability reduction and in development, or negative, resulting in a series of crises and emergencies, as well as setbacks in development initiatives.

Vulnerability to emergencies and disasters is a function of the degree of exposure to hazards and of people's capacity to cope with hazards and their consequences.[1] Community vulnerability has two aspects: susceptibility, the degree to which a community is exposed to hazards, and resilience, the community's capacity to cope with hazards. It is possible for a community to have either high or low susceptibility and resilience.

For example, many communities are susceptible to frequent severe earthquakes because of their geographical position and geological environment, while others do not experience them. Of the susceptible communities, some, like San Francisco, and many communities in Japan, are highly resilient and some, like Armenia, less resilient. This difference in resilience can be due to:

— different abilities of buildings, and various elements of the infrastructure, to withstand seismic loads;
— differences in emergency preparedness (i.e. the degree to which a community is organized to cope with emergencies);
— the extent of the resources that can be applied to an emergency;
— the degree to which the province or nation can sustain economic and social damage.

The vulnerability of units smaller and larger than a community, such as individual buildings, organizations, national economies, and political structures, can also be described in terms of susceptibility and resilience.

Vulnerability reduction requires a number of coordinated activities, including:

— policy development;
— vulnerability assessment (to describe the problems and opportunities);
— emergency prevention and mitigation (to reduce susceptibility);
— emergency preparedness (to increase resilience).

Without vulnerability assessment, communities will not know in what way they are vulnerable and how hazards may affect them. Without emergency prevention or mitigation, communities are exposed to unnecessary risk. Without emergency preparedness and response mechanisms, an emergency can escalate into a disaster, causing great harm and setting development back years. These aspects of vulnerability should all be addressed by any national policy (see Fig. 6).

Vulnerability assessment, also known as "hazard analysis" and "risk assessment", is based on a series of techniques for determining the hazards that may affect a particular community, and the impact they may have. It also determines what factors make the community vulnerable to emergencies and disasters, by

---

[1] Vulnerability is different from "vulnerable groups", such as the aged, women, children, the sick, and the poor. An assessment of vulnerability may identify and describe vulnerable groups, but this is only part of the overall picture. Vulnerable groups have differing degrees of susceptibility and resilience, and exist within the context of communities that themselves have differing degrees of susceptibility and resilience.

Fig. 6. **Vulnerability reduction**

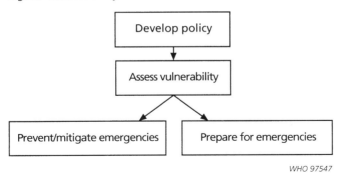

Fig. 7. **Number of cases of malaria following Hurricane Flora, Haiti, 1963**[a]

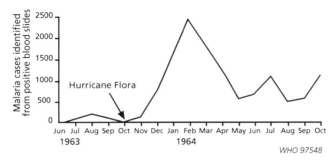

[a] Adapted from reference 5.

analysing the community's social, infrastructural, economic, and demographic composition.

Emergency prevention and mitigation involve measures designed either to prevent hazards from causing emergencies or to lessen the likely effects of emergencies. These measures include flood mitigation works, appropriate land-use planning, improved building codes, and relocation or protection of vulnerable populations and structures.

Emergency preparedness requires that emergency plans be developed, personnel at all levels and in all sectors be trained, and communities at risk be educated, and that these measures be monitored and evaluated regularly.

For example, Fig. 7 shows the prevalence of malaria before and after a hurricane. Malaria is just one of the health aspects of this emergency, and health is just one of the sectors affected. Emergency preparedness is required in the health sector to deal with the rapid changes in environment and disease brought about by emergencies.

A lack of preparedness will strain medical services and may ultimately impair development through increased morbidity and mortality in the population.

Because communities may be vulnerable to a broad range of hazards, the all-hazards approach should also be adopted. This approach entails developing strategies for all of the needs created by different types of potential emergencies. Each possible hazard can cause similar problems in a community, and actions such as warning, evacuation, mobilization of medical services, and assistance with community recovery may be required during and following emergencies. Thus, emergency preparedness can be based on common strategies and systems for the many different types of emergencies and disasters that might harm a community.

Certain hazards are of neither natural nor technological origin. Many forms of social exclusion can lead to social unrest, economic disruption, and violence. Such social exclusion may be caused by marginalization of the poor, tension between different ethnic and cultural groups, and other social inequities. One of the primary aims of development programmes with an integrated emergency preparedness component is to defuse potentially explosive social situations, and ensure the safety and security of the community.

Thus, vulnerability reduction addresses susceptibility by dealing with the causes of emergencies and disasters, and resilience, by strengthening communities that are still at risk.

Vulnerability reduction and development

Just as inappropriate humanitarian assistance can increase vulnerability, so vulnerability reduction can protect and enhance development. But how are vulnerability, hazards, and emergencies related to development?

It has been said that the purpose of development is to broaden people's range of choices. At the heart of this concept are three essential components:

— equality of opportunity for everyone in society;
— sustainability of opportunity from one generation to the next;
— empowerment of people so that they participate in and benefit from development processes (6).

Vulnerability to hazards is not spread equally throughout communities, and vulnerability reduction thus helps ensure equality of opportunity by reducing the susceptibility to harm of vulnerable groups. Emergencies are a direct threat to development, diverting development money to humanitarian assistance and damaging the structures that assist development. Vulnerability reduction is, like development, a process of empowering communities to take control of their own destinies.

Investing in vulnerability reduction protects human development achievements. Emergency preparedness also helps stricken communities limit the consequences of major emergencies and overcome them at an early stage, allowing development to resume.

Figure 8 illustrates how prepared communities can maintain and improve their level of development, despite emergencies. A prepared community will react to a potential disaster effectively, perhaps limiting it to the level of an emergency.

Fig. 8. **The effects of disasters on the development of prepared and unprepared communities**

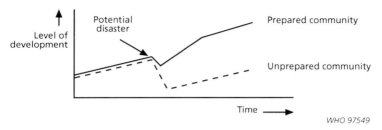

Fig. 9. **Emergency management cycle**[a]

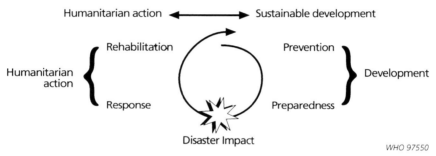

Note: Emergency management and development are linked. Prevention and preparedness measures should be integrated into development planning, in order to minimize the disaster impact. Response and rehabilitation are humanitarian activities which should contribute to sustainable development. Emergency management is a continuing process which is relevant not only at the time of the disaster impact, but also as an integral part of sustainable development.
[a] Reproduced from reference 7.

Thus, although the event may affect community development, its impact will be tempered. An unprepared community, however, may take years to recover from a severe setback in development.

Preparedness is a feature of many successful organizations in the world today. When a new or existing programme in an organization is being assessed, the risks, costs, and benefits are analysed. This allows the organization to ensure that its investment is protected, leading to a more secure future. These risk-management practices can be applied to communities: vulnerability reduction and emergency preparedness components should be built in to each new development, and whenever existing developments are reviewed (see Fig. 9).

The comprehensive approach combines prevention (and mitigation), preparedness, response, and recovery (rehabilitation). It is important that all sectors and organizations are active in each of these areas.

The responsibility for vulnerability reduction

Vulnerability reduction is often perceived as the exclusive domain of one organization, sector, or level of society and government. But a disaster — by definition

Fig. 10. **Vertical and horizontal integration of vulnerability reduction**

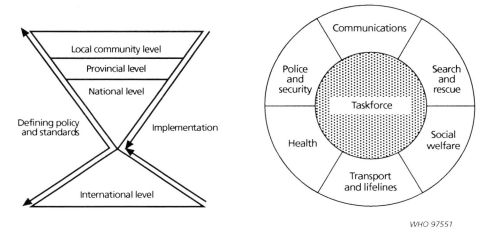

— exceeds the coping capacity of an entire community, and no single sector can manage vulnerability. Therefore, vulnerability reduction must be integrated into every sector of a country at every level — government, the private sector, and nongovernmental organizations (NGOs) — that is, both vertically and horizontally. Policy and standards for vulnerability reduction should come from the national level but implementing the various measures should begin at the community level (see Fig. 10). Six sectors at each administrative level should be involved in implementation, with a representative task force to coordinate the work. These sectors are: communications, health, police and security, search and rescue, social welfare, and transport and "lifelines".

Other sectors, such as education and environment should be included as appropriate, bearing in mind that vulnerability reduction must be integrated within the political and administrative context of each country.

The most successful management system for emergencies and disasters will be multisectoral and intersectoral. The multisectoral and intersectoral approach is one in which all organizations — government, private, and community — are involved in emergency management. Emergency management may entail different priorities for specific organizations (8), including:

— protecting their own interests and personnel;
— protecting the community from hazards arising from the activities of the organization;
— providing a public service to protect the community from likely hazards.

However, the emergency management work of each organization must be brought under a single, coordinated umbrella. If this approach is not applied, emergency management becomes fragmented and inefficient (7). The multisectoral and intersectoral approach will also help link emergency management to development, by institutionalizing emergency management and the use of its principles in development projects.

A key aspect of the multisectoral approach is that emergency management neither duplicates normal government administration nor acts independently of government. The control of government organizations should not be considered except in exceptional emergency circumstances.

In particular, it is imperative that organizations are not limited to the areas of emergency management in which they seem most active. So-called "response" and "relief" organizations should participate in all aspects of emergency management, including vulnerability assessment, prevention, mitigation, and preparedness.

Despite governmental and organizational involvement in emergency management, the community link remains the most critical one. Policy and standards must be defined by the national government, but communities should be allowed to develop and implement their own vulnerability reduction and emergency preparedness programmes because they will be the first to respond to emergencies. Provincial and national levels will support communities in their work, and the national government will provide the connection with international organizations and other countries.

Community emergency preparedness

The need for community-level emergency preparedness is illustrated by the live rescue rates following the Great Hanshin-Awaji (Kobe) earthquake of 17 January 1995 (see Fig. 11). Sixty-five percent of live rescues were accomplished in the first 24 hours. Within the first 3 days, the Kobe Fire Department had made 86% of their live rescues (9). Similarly, in the 1988 Armenian earthquake, 65% of the live rescues were made within the first 18 hours (10).

Only those in the immediate vicinity of an emergency or disaster, i.e. community members, can respond quickly and effectively. A community prepared for emer-

Fig. 11. **Live rescues made by the Kobe Fire Department following the Great Hanshin-Awaji (Kobe) earthquake**[a]

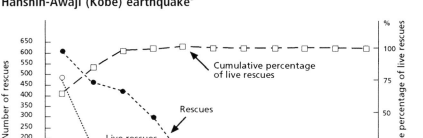

WHO 97552

[a] Reproduced from reference 9 by permission of the publisher.

gencies can rescue people rapidly and provide life-saving first aid: reliance on external assistance will lead to greater loss of life and harm to the community.

Because the community provides initial rescue and first aid, its capabilities should never be underestimated and with effective emergency preparedness these can be used to their utmost.

> "It is the victims of disaster who take action first to protect their lives, whether digging a neighbour out of the rubble after an earthquake or sifting through the city garbage to find things to sell and food to eat when drought turns grinding poverty into famine. If disaster relief is to be successful, it must build upon this tenacity for survival, working in partnership with, not imposing upon, the disaster victims." (*11*)

It has been shown that mortality rates in some types of emergencies can be reduced by 10% by simply placing the injured in the "lateral safety" or "coma" position. External humanitarian assistance may arrive too late, and may not be appropriate. If preparedness measures are taken seriously, families and the whole community will learn this type of self-reliance.

Local communities are at the centre of immediate response and recovery activities. Empowering local authorities to reduce a community's vulnerability and increase preparedness makes the most effective use of its action. Every level of government and each organization should support communities in this work, through the multisectoral approach.

The individuals in a community are responsible for maintaining its well-being. External assistance may be expected but it should not be relied on. Community members, resources, organizations, and administrative structures should be the cornerstones of an emergency preparedness programme. Listed below are some reasons that communities should prepare for emergencies (*7, 11*):

- Members of a community have the most to lose from being vulnerable to disasters and the most to gain from an effective and appropriate emergency preparedness programme.
- The positive effects of preparedness programmes can be best measured at the community level.
- Resources are most easily pooled at the community level and every community possesses capabilities. Failure to exploit these capabilities is poor resource management.
- Those who first respond to an emergency come from within a community. When transport and communications are disrupted, an external emergency response may not arrive for days.
- Sustained development is best achieved by allowing emergency-affected communities to design, manage, and implement internal and external assistance programmes.
- Excessive or inappropriate external assistance can destroy self-reliance and normal social and economic patterns, as well as increase both vulnerability and dependence on provincial, national, and international organizations.

This does not mean that each community should introduce a disaster management programme. Most communities are adequately prepared to deal with the harm caused by minor emergencies because experience has taught them to establish the necessary systems and resources. Existing routine emergency experience, organization, and resources can be built on to create disaster management preparedness.

Emergencies arise every day worldwide. An emergency can be defined as:

> "A sudden occurrence demanding immediate action that may be due to epidemics, to natural or technological catastrophes, to strife or to other man-made causes." (3)

Emergency management strategies can be used to prevent and respond to disasters. Methods for coping with severe road traffic accidents can be adapted to disaster rescue and medical services. The emergency management infrastructure can be employed to manage potential disasters since disasters are but the extreme end of the spectrum of harmful events.

> "Disasters are an extreme example of normal processes. The normal seasonal hunger turns into famine, the normal annual flood reaches its 20-year high point and the normal rise and fall of economic fortune plummets into economic collapse." (11)

Emergency management systems and strategies can be used to prevent disasters, despite limited resources for such activities, by better organizing established community resources and building on existing capabilities.

What is emergency preparedness?

Emergency preparedness is:

> "a programme of long-term development activities whose goals are to strengthen the overall capacity and capability of a country to manage efficiently all types of emergency and bring about an orderly transition from relief through recovery, and back to sustained development." (3)

The development of emergency preparedness programmes requires that the community's vulnerability be considered in context. Emergency preparedness can be ensured by creating a supportive political, legal, managerial, financial, and social environment to coordinate and use efficiently available resources to:

— minimize the impact of hazards on communities;
— coordinate an efficient transition from emergency response to recovery, according to existing goals and plans for development.

Thus, emergency preparedness and emergency management do not exist in a vacuum. To succeed, emergency preparedness programmes must be appropriate to their context. This context will vary from country to country and from community to community, but some relevant aspects are shown in Fig. 12.

There are a number of aspects to any management activity; in the context of emergency preparedness programmes they are:

INTRODUCTION

Fig. 12. **The context of emergency preparedness**[a]

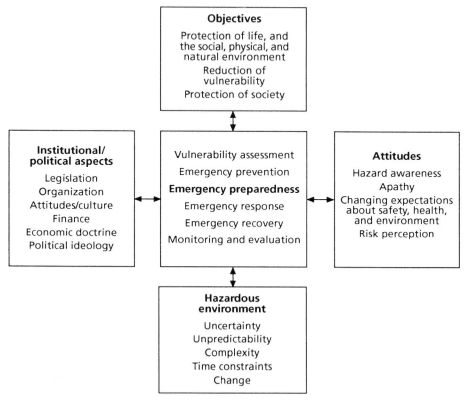

[a] Reproduced from reference *12* by permission of the publisher.

— content (the elements of an emergency preparedness programme);
— form (what the emergency preparedness programme looks like, and how it fits into real life);
— principles (the criteria used when making decisions about emergency preparedness);
— process (the methods used to develop preparedness).

Emergency preparedness includes the following elements:

— legal frameworks and enabling policy for vulnerability reduction;
— the collection, analysis, and dissemination of information on vulnerability;
— strategies, systems, and resources for emergency response and recovery;
— public awareness;
— organizational and human resource development.

These elements should be developed at community, provincial, and national levels. A capacity in each of these elements is a precondition for effective response and recovery when an emergency or disaster strikes. Without these elements, there will be no link between emergency preparedness and efficient emergency response on the one hand and recovery and development on the other. Developing and implementing an emergency preparedness programme will also produce significant secondary gains in encouraging local political commitment, community awareness, and intersectoral cooperation.

The basic principles of emergency preparedness are outlined below:

- It is the responsibility of all.
- It should be woven into the context of community, government, and NGO administration.
- It is an important aspect of all development policy and strategies.
- It should be based on vulnerability assessment.
- It is connected to other aspects of emergency management.
- It should concentrate on process and people rather than documentation.
- It should not be developed in isolation.
- It should use standard management techniques.
- It should concentrate not only on disasters but on integrating prevention and response strategies into any scale of emergency.

The process of preparing for an emergency (see Fig. 13) is a series of related methods for preparing a community, an organization, or an activity for emergencies. Each part of the process is explained briefly below (and most are discussed in greater detail in subsequent chapters).

Policy development (Chapter 2) includes developing emergency management legislation, normally established by a national government. It will mainly relate to the responsibility for emergency preparedness and special emergency powers.

Fig. 13. **An emergency preparedness process**

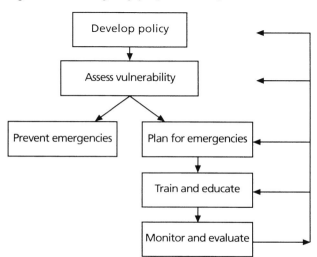

There is also a need for provincial and community organizations to develop policy relating to their specific geographical area. Similarly, private organizations and NGOs with emergency management responsibilities should develop appropriate policy in full partnership and consultation with the local authorities.

Vulnerability assessment (Chapter 3) can be used to identify those parts of a community that are vulnerable and in what ways; hazards that may affect a community and how they affect it; factors that render a community vulnerable and how vulnerability may be reduced; and the hazards that should be considered for emergency prevention and preparedness. Vulnerability assessment is also useful for response and recovery and for prevention and preparedness. It can be used to suggest areas that may have sustained damage and assist in assessing harm to the affected community, and provide a baseline for recovery and development strategies, by describing the "normal" state of a community.

Emergency prevention is based on vulnerability assessment and concerns the technical and organizational means of reducing the probability or consequences of emergencies, and the community's vulnerability. Emergency planning (Chapter 4) consists of determining:

— response and recovery strategies to be implemented during and after emergencies;
— responsibility for these strategies;
— the management structure required for an emergency;
— the resource management requirements.

Training and education (Chapter 5) concern training personnel in every aspect of emergency management and apprising the community of the kinds of hazards and the actions that may be required during emergencies, and the ways in which it can participate in emergency management.

Monitoring and evaluation (Chapter 6) determine how well the preparedness programme is being developed and implemented, and what needs to be done to improve it. Monitoring and evaluation are continuous processes, and any conclusions drawn should be included in policy development, vulnerability assessment, emergency management, and training and education.

Each section of this emergency preparedness process can be followed sequentially, but in practice, policy, vulnerability assessment, and emergency plans are often developed simultaneously. All of these activities should, however, be linked to ensure proper coordination.

Community participation

A community is composed of a group of people and the environment that supports them. For the purposes of this manual, a community will be defined as the people and environment contained at a local political and administrative level. This level needs to be small enough to allow community participation but there must be sufficient resources to permit realistic planning. Often planning will take place at several political or administrative levels simultaneously.

Because this manual is intended to be used in different countries, the following generic framework for government and administration has been assumed:

— community (the lowest administrative level within a country, corresponding to a village and its environs, county, town, or district);
— province (corresponding to a region or state);
— country (the national level).

Factors that may be relevant in assessing the vulnerability of a community and the ways in which it can recover from emergencies are demography, social structure, culture, economy, infrastructure, and environment. What is missing from these factors is the feeling of common interest, the social networks, and the shared experiences that exist within a community. Since communities are groups of individuals, most of whom need social interaction, there are many emotional and other mutual bonds between community members. These bonds form networks that may be difficult to analyse. They are, however, a very meaningful part of a community and play a significant role in its well-being.

There are also interactions between communities — the result of social, economic, or cultural ties. Thus, communities are not isolated but interconnected in a variety of ways. The effects of an emergency on a community will therefore be felt outside its strict administrative boundaries.

If one of the main principles of community emergency preparedness is community participation, how can this participation be ensured? Community participation should achieve the following:

— promote community awareness and education to reduce vulnerability and increase preparedness;
— allow the use of local knowledge and expertise, provide opportunities for participating in decisions that concern the community, and ensure policies and practices that allow for self-determination and maximum community involvement in response and recovery planning;
— ensure cooperation between professional personnel and volunteer members of the community;
— make use of the existing structures, resources, and local networks wherever possible, and of the community's own material and physical resources, particularly local suppliers;
— allow national and international organizations to channel resources directly to the community through predetermined and agreed procedures.

WHO describes community participation in the following ways:

> "*Marginal, substantive and structural participation.* Participation can be characterized in terms of three stages: marginal, substantive, and structural. . . . In marginal participation, community input is "limited and transitory and has little direct influence on the outcome of the development activity". Substantive participation is characterized by the community being actively involved in determining priorities and carrying out activities, even though the mechanisms for these activities may be externally controlled. In structural participation, the community is involved as an integral part of the

project and its participation becomes the ideological basis for the project itself. In this latter case, the community plays an active and direct part in all aspects of the development process and has the power to ensure that its opinions are taken into account.

Spontaneous, induced or compulsory participation. Experience has also demonstrated that participation can be characterized as spontaneous, induced or compulsory. In general, "spontaneous" participation refers to local initiatives which have little or no external support and which, from the very beginning, have the power to be self-sustaining. "Induced" participation, which appears to be more common, results from initiatives which are external to the community and which seek community support or endorsement for already defined plans or projects. "Compulsory" participation usually implies that people are mobilized or organized to undertake activities in which they have had little or no say, and over which they have no control.

Cooperation and power-sharing. Participation can also be classified on the basis of whether government is actively seeking cooperation or wishes to promote power-sharing. Where cooperation is sought, people are usually granted the right to receive information, to protest, to make suggestions and to be consulted before decisions are implemented. In power-sharing, the community is understood to have the right to share in all decision-making and has the power to veto ideas that are not in line with its own objectives."[1]

It should not, however, be assumed that a community represents a unified point of view. Often there are major conflicts of interest and the most vulnerable community members are excluded from decision-making. Real community participation requires methods for actively involving even the most marginalized community members, e.g. the disabled, homeless and displaced individuals, immigrants, and — in some societies — women.

The multisectoral, intersectoral, and all-hazards approach should be a partnership of relevant organizations and sections of the community, based on identifying vulnerabilities and planning action to reduce them. Within this framework, each partner accepts the responsibilities for which it is mandated, but within objectives defined by the community.

Project management

Whether for developing and implementing an entire emergency preparedness programme or for conducting a vulnerability assessment or emergency planning project, project management methods are often required. These methods are used to ensure that the project is:

— appropriate (it sets out to do something worthwhile);
— effective (it achieves the required results);
— efficient (it is completed on time and with the available resources).

---

[1] *Community action for health.* Geneva, World Health Organization, 1994 (background paper for 47th World Health Assembly, May 1994).

Project management methods are not an end in themselves and project management should not take over a project. Any project has a series of inputs and processes that produce outputs, which result in outcomes.

Inputs include people's time and energy; their perceptions of vulnerability and of emergency management requirements; money and resources; and commitment and perseverance. Processes, in this instance, are the processes of emergency preparedness. Outputs include:

— an understanding of the hazards and their likely effects;
— a community that is aware of these hazards and of its vulnerability;
— people who are aware of their responsibilities in emergency prevention, preparedness, response, and recovery;
— commitment to an emergency plan;
— enhanced emergency preparedness.

The outcomes of appropriate and effective emergency preparedness are the improved protection of life, property, and the environment, and the ability to sustain development.

There are three major parts to project management: project definition; project planning; and project implementation (*13*). These are described in Annex 1.

Summary

- Globally, the number of disasters is increasing with growing community vulnerability.
- Inappropriate humanitarian assistance can lead to reduced development assistance, increased community vulnerability, and further social crisis.
- Community vulnerability is a function of susceptibility and resilience.
- Vulnerability reduction can decrease the risk of emergencies and disasters by:
  — decreasing susceptibility (emergency prevention and mitigation);
  — increasing resilience (emergency preparedness).
- Vulnerability reduction also requires policy development and vulnerability assessment.
- Vulnerability reduction can protect and enhance development.
- Emergency management can be described by:
  — the comprehensive approach;
  — the all-hazards approach;
  — the multisectoral and intersectoral approach.
- The aims of civil protection, humanitarian action, and emergency management are very similar, and the same preparedness processes can be used for each. The health sector plays a key role, regardless of the system adopted by a country.
- Emergency preparedness is required at every level within a country, particularly at the community level.
- Community participation in emergency preparedness is essential for its success.
- Emergency preparedness processes can be used for any community, organization, or activity.

- Emergency preparedness should be developed to suit the context of the community.
- An emergency preparedness programme should be guided by project management methods.

References

1. International Federation of Red Cross and Red Crescent Societies. *World disasters report, 1993.* Dordrecht, Netherlands, Martinus Nijhoff, 1993.

2. *Bericht über das 116. Geschäftsjahr 1. Juli 1995 bis 30. Juni 1996. [Report for the 116th year of business 1st July 1996 to 30th June 1996.]* Munich, Münchener Rückversicherungs-Gesellschaft [Munich Reinsurance], 1996.

3. *Coping with major emergencies — WHO strategy and approaches to humanitarian action.* Geneva, World Health Organization, 1995 (unpublished document WHO/EHA/95.1, available from Emergency and Humanitarian Action, World Health Organization, 1211 Geneva 27, Switzerland).

4. Borton J. Recent trends in the international relief system. *Disasters*, 1995, 17(3):187–201.

5. Guha-Sapir D. Rapid assessment of health needs in mass emergencies: review of current concepts and methods. *World health statistics quarterly*, 1991, 44(3):171–181.

6. *Human development report.* New York, United Nations Development Programme, 1995.

7. *From disaster management to sustainable development: how the public sector, private sector and voluntary organizations can work together.* [World Conference on Natural Disaster Reduction, Main Committee Session, 1994, Yokohama, Japan.] Geneva, World Health Organization, 1994 (unpublished document WHO/EHA/EPP/Conf.94.4, available from Emergency and Humanitarian Action, World Health Organization, 1211 Geneva 27, Switzerland).

8. *National emergency management: competency standards.* Canberra, Emergency Management Australia, 1995.

9. Hayashi H, Kawata Y. Emergency and societal impacts of Great Hanshin-Awaji earthquake disaster of 17 January, 1995. In: *Proceedings of Third International Conference on Emergency Planning and Disaster Management, Lancaster, UK, 1995.* Preston, England, Lancaster City Council, 1995.

10. Noji EK et al. The 1988 earthquake in Soviet Armenia: a case study. *Annals of emergency medicine*, 1990, 19(8):891–897.

11. International Federation of Red Cross and Red Crescent Societies. *World disasters report, 1994.* Dordrecht, Netherlands, Martinus Nijhoff, 1995.

12. Parker D. The mismanagement of hazards. In: *Hazard management and emergency planning: perspectives on Britain.* London, James & James, 1992.

13. *Project management.* Princeton, NJ, Kepner-Tregoe, 1987.

Chapter 2
Policy development

Policy

Policy is "the formal statement of a course of action". Policy development is usually a "top-down" process, in that the central authority will prepare policy, and further decentralized policies may then be required. Policy is strategic in nature and performs the following functions:

— establishes long-term goals;
— assigns responsibilities for achieving goals;
— establishes recommended work practices;
— determines criteria for decision-making.

Policy is required to ensure that common goals are pursued within and across organizations, and that common practices are followed. Without agreed policies, efforts are fragmented, leading to lack of coordination and poor results.

While policies tend to be "top-down" (that is, authorized by higher levels), implementation of the strategies that arise from a policy tends to be "bottom-up", with higher levels assisting lower levels. Policy may also be created at all administrative levels of an organization or country, and be developed in consultation with those who are required to implement it. This ensures that a policy is realistic and achievable, and gains the commitment of those responsible for its implementation. Policy must be monitored and evaluated, and possibly revised. Specific responsibility for this should be allocated and evaluation criteria established.

Emergency preparedness policy

Policy development in relation to emergency preparedness can be broken down into principles, form, content, and process.

The emergency preparedness policy principles recognize the following (*1*):

- the rights of individuals and collective rights;
- the nature of the hazards, community, and vulnerability in the geographical area covered by the policy;
- existing related policies, including development, health, and environmental policy;
- existing legislative and organizational responsibilities;
- resource limitations;
- accepted emergency management concepts, including:
  — the comprehensive approach;
  — the all-hazards approach;
  — incorporating emergency preparedness into development planning;

- developing emergency management capabilities at the community level;
- community participation in emergency preparedness;
- building upon existing emergency capabilities;
- the multisectoral and intersectoral approach;
- public attitudes.

The form of emergency preparedness policy will vary both from country to country and between provinces in a given country. Policy may consist of community agreements, sectoral or intersectoral agreements, a provincial government decision, a national government executive decision, or legislation. The form should, however, maximize multisectoral participation. It is essential to emergency preparedness that all relevant organizations and levels are consulted to ensure joint commitment to community safety and well-being.

One process for emergency preparedness policy development is outlined below:

- A decision is made that policy is required and policy development is authorized.
- A qualified person (with a knowledge of policy development and emergency preparedness) is selected as the policy process manager.
- The policy process manager analyses the environment, culture, and administration of the area under his or her jurisdiction.
- A multisectoral team is selected to represent all of the organizations with an interest in emergency preparedness.
- The policy process manager and policy team consider the various emergency preparedness policy issues and document their decisions.
- The decisions on policy directions are publicized and debated in as many forums as possible.
- Final decisions on policy are made and formalized by the appropriate authorities (national legislature, national executive, provincial government, etc.).
- Policy is disseminated widely.

The next section, on emergency management policy, covers some of the options and questions on issues in emergency preparedness policy. It is suggested that the policy process manager does not give these lists of options and questions to the policy team. Rather, she or he should use them to prepare for policy development within the specific country context. The issues are summarized in the left-hand column of Table 1, with the recommended options shown in the right-hand column.

These policy issues may create considerable discussion and even disagreement among those responsible for emergency management, and countries and communities can choose any of numerous options to address them. The issues are detailed below, with options and discussion questions that can be used as a guide to policy and planning decision-making.

Issues in emergency management policy

The options and discussion questions below are meant only for the policy process manager to help him or her to be prepared for policy development meetings, and guide the process to reach the recommendation listed in Table 1.

Table 1. **Policy issues and recommended options**

Policy issue	*Recommended option*
1. Emergency preparedness and development planning	Emergency preparedness should be incorporated into all sustainable development objectives and projects.
2. National emergency law and other relevant enabling legislation	A national emergency law is required with references to emergency management in other laws. Definition of "emergency" should be broad, and the language of the law should be as simple as possible.
3. National emergency management organization	A national emergency management organization that is separate from other government agencies is preferable. Responsibility should also be decentralized to provincial government.
4. Responsibility and major mission of national emergency management organization	The mandate of the national organization, and its provincial counterparts, should cover all aspects of emergency management, including health.
5. Tasks of the emergency management organization	The organization should institutionalize emergency management in other organizations rather than attempt to undertake all emergency management work itself. It should undertake a number of tasks, but maintain a generalist approach.
6. Community and provincial emergency preparedness	The national level should develop policy and standards for emergency preparedness at all levels of government. Provincial and community-level emergency preparedness should be developed according to the policy and standards.
7. Health sector emergency preparedness	Health sector emergency preparedness should be coordinated with other sectors, the national level developing policy and standards, and the provincial and community levels implementing programmes. Public, private, military, and NGO health-service providers should be part of the same preparedness programme, as should each discipline within the health sector.
8. Involving other groups and citizens in emergency management	All citizens should be involved in emergency management in some way, ranging from active participation in vulnerability assessment and emergency planning, to receiving information on emergency preparedness.
9. Managing resources	Resources for emergency management should be based on existing resources. Emphasis should be on training and information-sharing in emergency management in all sectors and at all levels.
10. Evaluating an emergency preparedness and response programme	Performance indicators for emergency management should be developed to suit the national, provincial, and community environments.
11. Priorities in implementing emergency preparedness	Priorities should be based on either expressed or actual needs. This will require at least basic research into vulnerability and immediate needs.

Emergency preparedness and development planning
Options
- Do not institute emergency planning; leave the situation as it is.
- Keep emergency planning and development planning separate.
- Incorporate emergency planning into development planning.
- Initiate separate emergency planning but coordinate it with development planning.

Discussion questions
- Why give emergencies, which are statistically infrequent, priority over other social needs?
- What are the advantages and disadvantages of each option?
- What does emergency planning mean? What does development planning mean? Which concept should be used and why?
- What are the goals and objectives of planning of any kind?
- How can emergency planning be linked to sustainable development?

A national emergency law and other enabling legislation
Options
- Do not pass a new law. The country or community (or both) has survived without such legislation.
- Pass a new law that deals with emergencies only.
- Pass a law that deals not only with emergencies, but all hazards, including chronic as well as sudden risks, war or military situations as well as civil problems, and so on.
- Keep the terms of the law short and general; do not make it long and detailed.
- Define emergencies in terms of physical agents (e.g. flood, cyclone, explosion) or in terms of social effects and vulnerability (e.g. casualties, property losses, social disruption).
- Indicate gradations of emergencies; distinguish between everyday emergencies, disasters, and catastrophes. Are the differences quantitative or qualitative or both? What is the value of these distinctions?

Discussion questions
- Should the passage of a law be the first step in emergency preparedness?
- What would be gained or lost by adopting one or other of the various options indicated?
- What political considerations should be taken into account in attempting to pass any emergency legislation?
- Should consideration be given to the purposes of and problems in making fine legal distinctions?
- Given the variable nature of emergencies, might it not be wise to leave a degree of ambiguity or obscurity in defining an "emergency"?

The national emergency management organization

Options
- Make the armed forces the national organization responsible for emergency management.
- Give the responsibility to a special policy planning group in the prime minister's office.
- Increase the authority of some existing ministry (such as developmental planning or the ministry in charge of the police) to undertake emergency management.
- Create a new, national-level cabinet position with emergency management responsibility.
- Create a separate independent agency directly responsible to the president.
- Pass a national law, but decentralize responsibility to an organization in each of the provincial governments.
- Have no national organization, but make emergency management a "bottom-up" responsibility, to be undertaken by groups at the community and provincial levels.
- Give the responsibility to an NGO already operating nationwide and emergency-oriented (e.g. the national Red Crescent or Red Cross Society).

Discussion questions
- Why is there a need for a formal organization?
- How important is its location in the governmental structure?
- What are the advantages and disadvantages of the different options?
- What might be the case for using an established group or creating a new one for emergency purposes?
- Should consideration be given to establishing an organization that is partly protected from political pressure?
- Should a national-level organization be composed exclusively of specialists with relevant skills; professionals in public administration; political appointees; a combination of various skills and backgrounds? How might the personnel be recruited? Might the higher levels be composed of political appointees and the rest of the staff obtained through civil service examinations?

Responsibility and major mission of the national emergency management organization

Options
- The organization should be responsible for all aspects of emergency management, prevention/mitigation, preparedness, response, and recovery.
- The organization, while responsible for all aspects of emergency management, should focus primarily on prevention/mitigation.
- The organization should deal only with prevention/mitigation.
- Equal emphasis should be placed on structural mitigation measures (i.e. physical measures such as building dams) and non-structural mitigation measures (i.e. social measures such as training governmental officials on appropriate land use patterns or building codes).

- Emergency management should look forwards rather than backwards, concentrating on preventing and mitigating possible future emergencies rather than looking at past problems.

Discussion questions
- Is it possible to focus, in a meaningful way, on only one aspect of emergency management? Is there a difference between prevention and mitigation? If so, what are the implications for emergency management?
- Is the distinction between structural and non-structural measures (which to some extent is a distinction between physical and social activities) a meaningful one? Are not all such measures fundamentally social in nature, in that they require informing people and teaching them to do the right things?
- Should thought be given to how to project future emergencies, especially since they are likely to be somewhat different from past ones?
- Should consideration also be given to the possible relationship between the organization's major mission and the infrastructure or personnel that might be required? (For instance, a focus on mitigation/prevention may require professional knowledge of land use, zoning, building codes, and construction practices.)

Tasks of the emergency management organization

Options
- The organization should be almost exclusively an emergency planning group.
- In addition to emergency management, the organization should have regulatory/supervisory tasks (such as ascertaining whether dams have been properly constructed or whether building inspectors have the appropriate emergency-relevant knowledge).
- The organization should be primarily concerned with emergency planning during normal times, but should also have operational or management tasks during national emergencies.
- The organization should have a very broad mission; it should undertake a wide variety of functions, including policy setting, planning, provision of resources, gathering of information, monitoring, operations, and training.

Discussion questions
- Is a planning focus likely to lead to emphasis on the production of documents rather than on the planning process itself?
- If multiple tasks are to be undertaken, is there a logical or practical priority ranking that can be assigned to them?
- Should the implications of having a one-mission versus a multiple-mission organization be explored?

Community and provincial emergency preparedness

Options
- No formal attention should be paid to creating lower-level counterpart preparedness; provincial and local community governments would be responsible for this initiative.

- Only national-level entities and tasks should be discussed and decided at the present time. A decision on whether lower-level preparedness ought to be examined should be made later.
- National-level and lower-level entities and preparedness should be developed in parallel and simultaneously.
- While national-level activities should be given first priority, the national emergency legislation should set forth activities at the provincial and local community level that might be developed later.

Discussion questions
- What would be the positive and negative consequences of having (or mandating) a multilevel structure and preparedness programme?
- To what extent should lower-level structures and preparedness be similar to or parallel those at the national level?
- What are the implications of a primarily urban-based agency trying to initiate emergency preparedness for a mostly rural population?

Health sector preparedness

Options
- The health sector does not prepare for emergencies.
- Preparations are made for emergencies, but each part of the health sector conducts its own preparedness programme.
- Health sector preparedness is not coordinated with other sectors.
- A national emergency management cell is established in the health sector, to develop policy and standards.
- The health sector responds to emergencies at the national level only.
- The provincial level of the health sector responds to emergencies, assisted by the national level.

Discussion questions
- How can the health sector fit in with multisectoral emergency preparedness?
- Who is responsible, within the health sector, for emergency preparedness and response?
- Should private, public, military, and nongovernment health providers coordinate their emergency preparedness programmes?
- What is the most efficient way of organizing health sector emergency preparedness?
- Does the ministry of health have the legislative power to coordinate emergency preparedness?
- How do community health organizations communicate with the national health level?
- Who is ultimately responsible for health sector emergency preparedness?

Involving other groups and citizens in emergency management

Options
- Others should not be formally involved.
- Only other government organizations should be involved.

POLICY DEVELOPMENT

- Besides the government, the private sector and NGOs should also be involved.
- There should be a selective involvement of key community officials.
- All citizens should be involved in emergency management in some way.
- All should be involved but there should be a definite sequencing for involvement in the planning process.

Discussion questions
- How is the credibility of emergency management to be established in government bureaucracies?
- Are there special problems in securing the involvement of industry and industrial workers in emergency management?
- Is it worth using national heroes, celebrities, and educational campaigns to increase citizens' awareness?
- What degree of citizens' involvement in any emergency management programme is there? What kind of involvement? For what reasons? Some argue that without extensive citizen participation (or at least interest), no meaningful emergency management programmes can be undertaken. Others argue that, strategically, it is best to start a programme with a core of key community officials or leaders.

Managing resources

Options
- There should be funding for institution-building and other community activities and entities relevant to emergency prevention.
- A cadre or core of specialists in emergency management should be quickly established.
- A full range of facilities and equipment (e.g. training centres, computers with appropriate software) should be provided for the emergency management organizations.

Discussion questions
- Should direct funding be provided for increasing and strengthening coping mechanisms for emergencies at the local community level?
- What are the advantages and disadvantages of sending officials abroad for training in emergency management?
- Should emergency training centres and programmes be developed within existing educational institutions or should new organizations be created?
- Is it easier to fund non-structural activities (e.g. training or educational programmes) than structural measures (e.g. building dams), since the latter often require considerable capital investment as well as maintenance costs?
- Should thought be given to whether information distribution and sharing should be considered as a resource allocation mechanism?

Evaluating an emergency preparedness and response programme

Options
- Set milestones and deadlines for meeting specific goals.
- Obtain feedback from citizens.

- Undertake research.
- Require periodic reports be made to the government.

Discussion questions
- Does a focus on deadlines, schedules, and reports lead to a concern with administrative matters rather than with the quality of what is being attempted?
- What are the relative advantages and disadvantages of having insiders (i.e. members of the organization involved) or outsiders evaluating a programme? Can candid and honest organizational self-assessments be obtained?
- Should there be an examination of the type of research and social science that would be most useful for emergency planners? What should be the relationship between researchers and emergency managers? Does an interest in applied research preclude supporting basic research?

Priorities in implementing emergency preparedness
Options
- A systematic national emergency vulnerability assessment is the highest priority.
- A mass information or educational campaign about emergency planning is necessary and should be given early priority.
- Priorities should be set in terms of the sectors that are most important in the society.

Discussion questions
- In what ways might symbolic activities (such as proclaiming a national emergency day, a public address on the topic by a senior figure, statements of support by well-known figures) be important first steps in initiating an emergency planning programme?
- Since everything cannot be done at once, should the easier tasks or those offering the greatest long-term advantage be undertaken first?
- How should the choice be made between planning for a likely emergency and planning for a more unlikely catastrophe?
- How will political considerations affect decision-making on setting of priorities?

Summary
- Policy is strategic in nature, concerns the establishment of long-term goals, assigns responsibilities for achieving goals, may establish recommended work practices, and may determine criteria for decision-making.
- Policy development is a process.
- Emergency management policy should be developed in line with accepted emergency management principles.
- Policy should be widely debated.
- Policy issues include:
  — emergency preparedness and development planning;
  — national emergency law and other relevant enabling legislation;

- national emergency management organization;
- responsibility and major mission of the national emergency management organization;
- tasks of the emergency management organization;
- community and provincial emergency preparedness;
- health sector emergency preparedness;
- involving other groups and citizens in emergency management;
- managing resources;
- evaluating an emergency preparedness and response programme;
- priorities in implementing emergency preparedness.

Reference

1. *National emergency management competency standards.* Canberra, Emergency Management Australia, 1995.

Chapter 3
Vulnerability assessment

Introduction
The value of vulnerability assessment
Vulnerability assessment (also known as "hazard analysis", "threat assessment", and "risk assessment") is a procedure for identifying hazards and determining their possible effects on a community, activity, or organization. It provides information essential for:

— sustainable development (because development will be undermined without programmes and strategies to reduce vulnerability);
— emergency prevention, mitigation, and preparedness (without knowledge of what is likely to go wrong, and what the effects will be, it is impossible to be effectively prepared and difficult to prevent problems);
— emergency response (many emergencies seriously disrupt transportation and communications, and information may become either unreliable or non-existent; vulnerability assessment will suggest where most of the damage might occur);
— emergency recovery (vulnerability assessment can provide a baseline that describes the prior condition of the community, against which the effectiveness of recovery work can be compared).

There are numerous ways of assessing vulnerability. The process described in this manual consists of a series of steps, each containing a number of techniques. Some of these steps are hazard identification, community and environmental analysis, and hazard description. In turn, there are techniques for identifying hazards, for describing the people, property, and environment they may affect, and for describing hazards.

The meaning of "vulnerability"
Vulnerability is the result of a number of factors that increase the chance that a community will be unable to deal with an emergency. Not all sections of a community are vulnerable to hazards, but most are vulnerable to some degree. Vulnerability comprises two aspects — susceptibility and resilience.

Susceptibility concerns the factors operating in a community that allow a hazard to cause an emergency; examples of such factors range from a community's level of development to its location in an earthquake-prone area.

Resilience is the community's ability to withstand the damage caused by emergencies and disasters; it is a function of the various factors that allow a community to respond to and recover from emergencies.

VULNERABILITY ASSESSMENT

Communities and the individuals of which they are composed have a number of general needs during and after emergencies, of which personal safety is the most obvious. Thus, caring for the injured and protecting people from further harm are of paramount importance, together with providing food, drink, and shelter.

The meaning of "hazard"

In emergency management, "hazard" has various definitions. This manual defines "hazard" as any phenomenon that has the potential to cause disruption or damage to people and their environment.

Other definitions within the context of emergency management include:

— a threat to people and what they value;
— a threat to life, well-being, material goods, and environment from the extremes of natural processes and technology;
— potential for an agent or process to do harm.

Common to all these definitions is the potential for harm. A hazard is not an event — it is the potential for an event. Thus "flood", in a general sense or even as applied to a particular place, is a hazard. An actual flood is an "incident", "emergency", or "disaster", depending on the damage it causes or how well it is managed. A vulnerability assessment relating to a flood in a particular community examines the potential for flood events and the possible effects of such events. Analysing a flood that has occurred is not a vulnerability assessment because each event is unique, and emergency management based on a specific event will contain too many unjustified assumptions. What is true of one flood will not necessarily be true of another.

Communities, environments, and hazards

In terms of emergency management, a community has an intimate relationship with its environment and its hazards. The following example illustrates how a community interacts with its environment and hazards. People move into a hilly, forested area, with a medium to high annual rainfall, and clear land for agriculture. Before the forest was cleared, rainfall was absorbed and trapped by vegetation and accumulated humus before it could run off into creeks and rivers. Forests and many other natural ecosystems, such as swamps, act as sponges during heavy rain by storing water, some of which then evaporates or is released slowly. While there is still the potential for flood, only the heaviest rain will cause serious flooding. Once a forested area is cleared, drainage characteristics change. There is less vegetation and humus to collect and store water, so the water runoff is greater. There is also more erosion, and the profile of the river bed is altered by the accumulation of silt. When heavy rainfall occurs, therefore, there is a greater likelihood of serious flooding, which may lead, in turn, to further changes in the drainage system.

If part of this community lives on or near flood plains, and the settlement took account only of the flood characteristics that existed before forest clearing, problems might occur, including:

— severe floods leading to loss of life and destruction of buildings, bridges, roads, dams, and livestock;

- removal of valuable topsoil from agricultural areas and, hence, decreasing productivity;
- river siltation, leading to changes in the navigability of the river.

Thus, changes in the environment caused by the community alter the hazards in the area, and the changed hazards may then have effects on the environment, the community, and the community's vulnerability. It is essential, therefore, to examine how the community, the environment, and the hazards interact when performing a vulnerability assessment.

Even normal population growth can increase vulnerability, by forcing communities into marginal and hazardous areas.

The process of vulnerability assessment

The purpose of the process

There are several reasons why a rational process for assessing vulnerability is needed:

- to explain to others what is being done and how they can participate;
- to ensure that significant aspects of the vulnerability assessment are not missed;
- to justify the validity of the results, demonstrating that analysis has been thorough (this is particularly important when funding for emergency management is sought).

The steps in this process should be followed consecutively and information from each step used in subsequent ones (see Fig. 14).

Parts of the process

The parts of the vulnerability assessment process are as follows:

- The *project definition* determines the aim, objectives, scope, and context of the vulnerability assessment, the tasks to be performed, and the resources needed to perform them. This is described in Annex 1.
- The formation of a representative *planning group* is essential to vulnerability assessment and emergency planning. Without this group it will be difficult to gather the required information, obtain the commitment of key individuals, and allow the community to participate.
- *Hazard identification* reveals the hazards that exist in the community (although it is unlikely that all of the hazards will be discovered).
- *Hazard description* presents the hazards that exist in the community. The same hazards may manifest themselves differently in different areas and communities because there is an interaction between hazards, the particular community, and the environment.
- A *community and environment description* outlines the relevant information about the people, property, or environment that may affect or be affected by the hazards. More hazards may be identified at this stage.
- A description of *effects* is an account of community vulnerability — what is likely to happen in an accident, incident, emergency, or disaster involving a single hazard or multiple hazards.

Fig. 14. **The vulnerability assessment process**

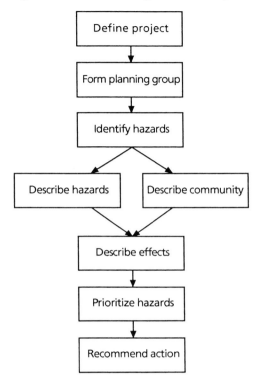

- *Hazard prioritization* determines the hazards that should be dealt with first, and those that can be dealt with later or ignored, on the basis of their likely effects and community vulnerability.
- *Recommendations for action* are the link between vulnerability assessment and other emergency management activities. Planning, training and education, and monitoring and evaluation should be based firmly on the results of the vulnerability assessment.
- *Documentation* of all results and decisions is necessary to justify the recommendations, and any further emergency preparedness work.

Some problems in assessing vulnerability

Some of the common problems encountered in performing vulnerability assessments relate to data, lack of knowledge, attitudes, project scope, and rigid adherence to the process.

- *Data* — Unavailability of data on some hazards; data of unknown reliability; too much data on other hazards; too much data on communities and difficulty in determining which are relevant.
- *Knowledge* — Lack of knowledge in the community or the planning group of the methods of vulnerability assessment; lack of knowledge of specific hazards.

- *Attitudes* — A lack of cooperation from some agencies, particularly response agencies, who may perceive vulnerability assessment as an academic exercise only.
- *Project scope* — Poor definition of the area covered by the vulnerability assessment; trying to analyse too much; determining the amount of detail required in the hazard and community descriptions; presenting unrealistic and unachievable recommendations.
- *Rigid adherence to process* — Forcing the hazard and community descriptions into too rigid a framework — some of the characteristics suggested in this manual will not work with some hazards and communities; following the process in a lock-step manner and not allowing a return to earlier steps when required.
- *Frustration with the process* — It is possible that the planning group and the community will become frustrated with the vulnerability assessment process (problem analysis) and want to start emergency planning (problem-solving). It may be possible to begin planning and implementing vulnerability reduction while a formal vulnerability assessment is being performed, but a complete vulnerability assessment remains desirable.

Alternative processes

The vulnerability assessment process described here — and the planning process described in Chapter 4 — is one way of analysing and solving emergency preparedness problems. Another approach, which can be used to help start more formal vulnerability assessment and emergency planning, is the "community needs and resource maps" method. This method encourages community participation at the grass roots by:

- encouraging people to describe their problems;
- developing a preliminary list of community risks and needs;
- using field visits to verify risks and needs, and then creating maps that illustrate the problems and the available resources;
- establishing a local committee to make plans to deal with the identified risks and needs.

While this method is useful, the formal processes of vulnerability assessment and emergency planning allow for a more accurate description of hazards and vulnerability and better emergency preparedness.

The planning group

Why a planning group is necessary

Once a project definition has been developed, forming a planning group is the second step in the vulnerability assessment process. Why is a planning group essential to the development of appropriate vulnerability assessments and emergency plans?

- Firstly, rapid access to diverse information is essential. It is possible to gather this information through correspondence, interviews, and telephone calls, but this will take time. Assembling the people who can provide information will make information-gathering more efficient.

- Secondly, no one is expert in everything and the contributions of experts in particular fields are required. Local experts may become the greatest critics of a vulnerability assessment if they are ignored.
- Lastly, if the vulnerability assessment is to be taken seriously, the commitment of all relevant personnel is essential. Allowing people to contribute to the vulnerability assessment objectives and to work together towards a common goal are effective means of gaining this commitment.

Before a planning group is selected it is important to find out whether one already exists. There may well be a group of people who are responsible for safety and crisis or emergency management in a given community. If such a group exists, it may be ideal for the purposes of preparing a vulnerability assessment because it may already have sufficient resources, the necessary authority, appropriate representation, an efficient reporting system, and sufficient expertise.

The suitability of any existing emergency management group should be assessed on the basis of the above criteria, as well as by reference to the project definition. Any shortcomings in the planning group will need to be addressed.

A planning group need not be fixed in its membership. The group will evolve according to its activities, and the end result will be a group of people committed to emergency preparedness in their community, who will be able to work together during actual emergencies. However, changes in the planning group composition, although desirable, may cause problems. Groups of people who work together will often develop a strong sense of unity and newcomers may often find it difficult to win the group's acceptance or feel comfortable working with it. Understanding this potential problem is already a partial solution; group members must welcome new members and avoid forming barriers between themselves and the community.

The planning group may also serve as a formalized emergency committee. Each member must therefore have sufficient authority to represent his or her organization in preparedness and response.

Working with the planning group

To work effectively with the planning group, the following should be considered. Firstly, the project definition will provide the group with a description of its aim, objectives, scope, and authority to take action. The group should be informed of the process for developing the vulnerability assessment. It will need to know the benefits of the assessment and the nature of the final product. The group will also need to understand how long the vulnerability assessment will take to develop and what resources will be used.

The following aspects of planning group meetings should be resolved:

— the authority of the group;
— the method of reporting;
— the means of communicating meeting dates and times;
— the frequency and timing of meetings;

— the conduct of meetings (chairing, agenda, minutes, recommendations, and follow-up actions);
— any educational requirements of the group.

It is essential that the planning group members discuss the project definition and make alterations if they see fit.

Once a planning group is assembled, it may be found that the individual members, coming from varied backgrounds and with different responsibilities in emergency management, have remarkably different perceptions of risk.

Risk perception

Risk perception is about the relationship between hazards, knowledge, and people's attitudes. It is impossible to be totally objective when assessing vulnerability or developing emergency plans, and so it is necessary to understand some of the different ways people approach the subject — they may have very different views on the nature and extent of the risk that a particular hazard presents, and on what constitutes vulnerability.

It is important to consider people's perceptions and attitudes in vulnerability assessment because these will strongly influence their actions. This inevitably leads to the question of whose perceptions of risk are right — and, indeed, whether there are right and wrong perceptions. Some may suggest that the opinions of experts in a given field must be correct, but such opinions are still based on individual perceptions. In addition, experts are not always exposed to the risks they are studying, unlike members of the community.

Table 2 shows some of the reasons for differences in risk perception between technical people and the general community.

Table 2. **Factors relevant to the technical and cultural attitudes to risk**[a]

Technical attitude	*Cultural attitude*
Trust in scientific methods, explanations and evidence	Trust in political culture and democratic process
Appeal to authority and expertise	Appeal to folk wisdom, peer group and traditions
Boundaries of analysis are narrow and reductionist	Boundaries of analysis are broad; includes use of analogy and historical precedent
Risks are depersonalized	Risks are personalized
Emphasis on statistical variation and probability	Emphasis on the impacts of risk on the family and community
Appeal to consistency and universality	Focus on the particularity; less concern about consistency of approach
Where there is controversy in science, resolution follows status	Popular responses to scientific differences do not follow prestige principle
Impacts that cannot be specific are irrelevant	Unanticipated or unarticulated risks are relevant

[a]Reproduced from reference 1 (© 1987 by Sage Publications, Inc.) by permission of the publisher.

People with technical training or inclinations will tend to view hazards and vulnerability in terms of abstract risk. Risk is often described by the likelihood of a given harm, for example the probability of fatality from a hazard. Table 3 illustrates some typical individual fatality risks.

The general public, however, which does not have access to the data that permit numerical calculations of the probability of harm, will tend to use factors like those shown in Table 4.

If a hazard is characterized by a number of the factors on the right-hand side of Table 4, the public is likely to perceive it as a serious problem. This is not an irrational response, but a response based upon people's feelings and experience.

Different people think about hazards and vulnerability in different ways, and may use different criteria for judging their seriousness. The uncertainties of risk and vulnerability preclude correct perceptions of risk, although some perceptions may be more realistic than others. It is important to understand people's perceptions in order to develop appropriate emergency management strategies and to work with a diverse planning group.

Table 3. **Risk to individuals**[a]

Hazard	Individual fatality risk level[b]	Hazard	Individual fatality risk level[b]
Smoking 10 cigarettes a day (UK)	5000×10^{-6}	Taking contraceptive pills	20×10^{-6}
Cancer (all causes — Australia)	1800×10^{-6}	Homicide (Australia)	20×10^{-6}
All natural causes, age 40 (UK)	1200×10^{-6}	Working in radiation industry (UK)	17.5×10^{-6}
Any kind of violence or poisoning (UK)	300×10^{-6}	Homicide (Europe)	10×10^{-6}
Influenza (UK)	200×10^{-6}	Floods (northern China)	10×10^{-6}
Accident on road (driving in Europe)	125×10^{-6}	Floods (USA)	2.2×10^{-6}
Accident at home (Australia)	110×10^{-6}	Accident on railway (Europe)	2×10^{-6}
Struck by motor vehicle (pedestrian — USA)	50×10^{-6}	Bushfire (Australia)	1×10^{-6}
Leukaemia	50×10^{-6}	Earthquake (California)	0.5×10^{-6}
Earthquake (Islamic Republic of Iran)	43×10^{-6}	Bites of venomous creatures (UK)	0.2×10^{-6}
Playing field sports (UK)	40×10^{-6}	Storm and flood (Australia)	0.2×10^{-6}
Accident at home (UK)	38×10^{-6}	Hit by lightning (UK)	0.1×10^{-6}
Accident at work (UK)	23×10^{-6}	Wind storm (northern Europe)	0.1×10^{-6}
Floods (Bangladesh)	20×10^{-6}	Rupture of pressure vessel (USA)	0.05×10^{-6}

[a] Reproduced from reference 2 by permission of the publisher. Copyright John Wiley & Sons Ltd.
[b] A fatality risk of 1×10^{-6} means that there is a 1 in 1 million chance of an individual being killed as a result of a particular hazard in any given year.

Table 4. **Factors relevant to hazards that may affect people's perception**[a]

Perceived as unimportant	Perceived as serious
Voluntary	Involuntary
Natural	Man-made
Familiar	Exotic
Not memorable	Memorable
Common	Dread
Chronic	Catastrophic
Controlled by individual	Controlled by others
Fair	Unfair
Morally irrelevant	Morally relevant
Detectable	Undetectable
Visible benefits	No visible benefits
Trusted source	Untrusted source

[a]Reproduced from reference 3 by permission of the authors.

Hazard identification
General
Hazard identification determines the hazards that may affect people in a community. This third step in the vulnerability assessment process provides information for further analysis. Hazard identification is not straightforward — people may have quite different perceptions of what constitutes a significant hazard. For this reason seeking the views of a number of people in the community is essential.

A group technique for identifying hazards
Hazard identification should be undertaken by a group of people, such as a planning group, with expertise in the area of work and a commitment to the safety of that area. One quick method to determine people's perceptions of the most serious hazards and avoid the pitfalls of "groupthink",[1] is the following:

- Each person in the group should be asked to write down the 10 hazards (in the area being investigated) that most concern them, and be given a few minutes to do this.
- When they have finished the first task, they should rank, in terms of "seriousness", the hazards they have listed as "high", "medium", and "low" (using their own definition of "seriousness").
- Each person should then say what he or she has written down (without the ranking) and answers should be recorded on a blackboard, whiteboard, or large sheet of paper. Duplications should not be recorded; if very similar hazards are mentioned, planning group members should refine what they mean. Suggestions must not be belittled, but recorded uncritically.
- When each person has contributed, a table similar to Table 5 should be drawn up.
- Group members should be asked about each hazard listed; the numbers of

---

[1] "Groupthink" is a phenomenon that can occur in highly cohesive groups — to minimize conflict, the members of the group concur and restrict their thinking to the norms of the group. No one wishes to be seen as out of place. This can limit the range of ideas and views that the group could otherwise generate.

Table 5. **Hazard ranking**

Hazard	In terms of "seriousness"		
	high	medium	low
Hazard "a"	2	3	0
Hazard "b"	0	0	1
Hazard "c"	4	0	1
Hazard "d"	0	2	0

people who consider each hazard to be high, medium, or low in seriousness should be recorded.

The numbers recorded in the table indicate how people in the planning group feel about the hazards in the community and may reflect accurate knowledge on their part. The numbers certainly reflect the group's perception of which hazards are a problem. The numbers have no meaning outside the context of the planning group meeting and certainly should not be used for any other purposes.

This technique has the following benefits.

- It allows everyone to have their say and avoids some of the problems of "groupthink". If everyone is allowed to contribute, the likelihood of developing a meaningful vulnerability assessment is greater.
- It encourages interaction between people who may not know each other and may encourage all group members to continue contributing.
- It prompts the members of the planning group to think analytically.
- It demonstrates to all members of the group that people have divergent points of view concerning hazard and risk and will to some extent validate these different points of view.
- It increases members' commitment to the vulnerability assessment because they have had a chance to contribute.

Other techniques for identifying hazards

Other techniques for identifying hazards include:

— researching the history of emergencies in the community, by consulting histories, newspapers, records, and older community members;
— inspecting the community for evidence of previous emergencies, existing hazards, and existing vulnerability;
— examining literature or interviewing people from similar communities;
— requesting information from provincial or national governments.

Hazard description

General

Five basic characteristics can be used to describe most hazards:

— intensity (how big, fast, and powerful);
— frequency (the likelihood of a hazard causing an event of a given magnitude);

— extent (the area that a hazard may affect);
— time frame (warning time, duration, time of day, week, year);
— manageability (whether anything can be done about it).

For each hazard, these characteristics may mean different things. In a cyclone, for example, intensity might relate to wind speed, whereas in an earthquake, intensity relates to the number and strength of earth tremors. The example in the following section deals with flooding.

Description of a flood hazard

Flood intensity
Flood intensity may be described by height, class, depth, flow rate, and speed.

Height. Flood height is often described in relation to a fixed marker, such as a post with heights marked on it, often placed in an arbitrary position near the river. Thus, a river height of 4 metres at one point on the river may be a fairly normal height, whereas the same height at a different place will indicate that the river is in flood.

Class. Floods may also be described in terms of classes. Definitions will vary from country to country, but the following are typical:

- Minor flooding — flooding that causes inconveniences, such as the closure of minor roads and the submergence of low-level bridges.
- Moderate flooding — low-lying areas are inundated, requiring the removal of livestock and evacuation of some houses; main traffic bridges may also be submerged.
- Major flooding — extensive rural areas are flooded, with properties and towns isolated; large urban areas are also flooded.

In flood warnings, both the heights and the flood classes are often given for different points on a river; local people who receive the warnings may use their prior experience of either description to decide how to act.

Depth. Another way of describing the intensity of floods is to relate flood heights to the floor levels of buildings that may be affected. This gives an idea of depth and is very useful for planning evacuation, land use, and building protection.

Flow rate. Flow rate describes the volume of water flowing past a particular point in a given time period, and the units are either cusecs (cubic feet per second) or cumecs (cubic metres per second), where 1 cusec = 0.028 cumecs, and 35 cusecs = 1 cumec. This method of description is often used in relation to dam safety, as a very high flow rate over a dam with insufficient spillway capacity may lead to dam failure.

Speed. Flood intensity may also be described in terms of the speed of the water at a given point. This is a useful measure since speed, coupled with water depth, will indicate the scale of damage of which the moving water is capable. Figure 15 shows the speed and depth of flowing water that can cause failure to various building types.

Fig. 15. **Critical flood speed and depth for building failure**[a]

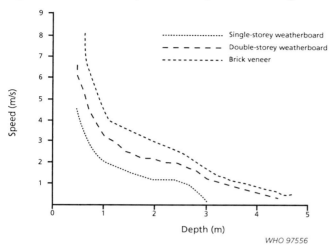

[a] Reproduced from reference 4 by permission of the publisher.

Table 6. **Flood frequency likelihood**

Definitions of average recurrence interval (ARI)	Definitions of annual exceedance probability (AEP)
(a) the average or expected value of the period between exceedances of a given discharge	(a) the probability of exceedance of a given discharge within a period of 1 year
(b) the expected time interval (usually in years) between floods of a given level	(b) the probability in any year that a flood of a given level will occur

Floods occurring in flat areas, where the water moves very slowly, are obviously less likely to cause structural damage.

Describing the speed of floodwater also makes it easier to determine when and where rescue boats can be used — boats will not make headway against water that is moving at the normal speed of the boat or faster.

Flood frequency or likelihood
Flood frequency or likelihood is often described in terms of average recurrence interval (ARI) and annual exceedance probability (AEP). These two terms are defined in Table 6 in two ways: (a) in strictly correct, engineering terms (5), and (b) less formally.

Annual exceedance probability is usually expressed in terms of "1 in 100", "1 in 50", etc. or of 1%, 2%, etc. chance of occurrence in any one year, and rivers may be described using a flood frequency curve, an example of which is shown in Fig. 16.

Fig. 16. **An example of a flood frequency curve**[a]

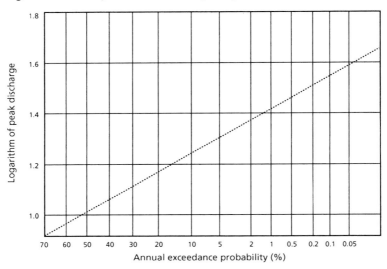

WHO 97557

[a] Reproduced from reference 5 by permission of the publisher.

The horizontal axis of the graph shows the annual exceedance probability as a percentage, and the vertical axis shows the logarithm of the peak flood discharge (in cumecs). The diagonal line is the flood frequency curve, which indicates the estimated or expected probability of a given discharge for this particular river. Taking one point on the curve, the probability of a peak discharge of 10 cumecs (shown as 1.0, i.e. $\log_{10} 10$; 100 cumecs would be shown as 2.0, i.e. $\log_{10} 100$) is about 50%. The flood frequency curve is based on data from a number of floods over a period of years. It is usual, however, for actual recorded flows or discharges to cluster above and below this line.

The means for describing flood frequency thus includes an element of the description of intensity (in this case, discharge in cumecs).

Flood extent
The extent of a flood is best described using a map. Some flood maps may be used to describe the flood hazard for an entire country, or they may detail particular sections of rivers. The more detailed flood maps should ideally show the following information:

- one or more historical major flood levels;
- the flood levels for a variety of annual exceedance probabilities, typically 5% (1/20), 2% (1/50), and 1% (1/100);
- some of the roads and structures and details of land use in the area;
- flood levels that are considered to represent minor, moderate, and major floods;
- flow rates at particular points in the river for given flood levels.

A table showing the major historical flood events, attached to the flood map, would also provide essential information in describing flood extent.

Flood time-frame
The time-frame of flooding refers to:

— how much warning time there is (the time-lag between detecting or predicting the flood and disseminating information about it);
— how much lead time there is (the period between receipt of the warning and action being taken);
— the time of year when floods are more likely to occur;
— the length of time over which the flood will continue to cause damage and hamper response efforts.

Flood manageability
Flood manageability is a measure of the degree to which floods can be prevented, prepared for, responded to, and recovered from. This will vary enormously from river to river and from area to area.

Conclusion
This description of flooding shows that some hazards can be described reasonably thoroughly. This is not true, however, of all hazards. When the characteristics of intensity, frequency, extent, time-frame, and manageability do not seem to fit a hazard or if they appear incomplete, analysis using an inappropriate model should not be attempted. If these characteristics do not suit the hazard, they should be removed, or new characteristics considered, as necessary. The descriptors used should be the most appropriate for the hazard.

Description of technological hazards
Technological hazards are caused by the processes and materials of life in an industrialized world. They include:

— the transport of people and materials (by road, rail, air, or sea);
— the use of heavy or fast-moving machinery;
— the use of high pressure, high temperature, electricity, etc;
— the manufacture, storage, use, and disposal of hazardous materials.

The reasons for performing industrial hazard analysis depend on the perspective of those involved, and are summarized in the following paragraphs.

The community, including some members of the government, expects industry to be completely "safe". Attitudes towards the safety of industry tend to differ from attitudes towards safety in other activities, such as driving and sports, and are often unrealistic. Often, certain industries are targeted, while other less safe ones are ignored. For example, the degree of concern about industries involved in radioactive-related activities may be disproportionate compared with concern about other types of industries.

Industries are under increasing pressure from the community and government to minimize the risk of employee accidents and larger hazardous events that could affect the community. One measure that allows them to appear responsible is to perform hazard analysis.

Hazard analysis, coupled with comprehensive safety systems, has the potential to increase the viability of industry. Those industries that are aware of the principles of risk management may have differing degrees of concern about the risks involved in their activities, and may see sufficient benefit from the risks posed to allow them to continue at their current levels, or may consider the cost of reducing the risks to be too high. Industries that are unaware of the degree of risk involved in their activities or of the principles of risk management would probably resist any expenditure on hazard analysis or comprehensive safety systems.

A wide variation in the degree of safety of different types of industry, and in the interest that industrial management would have in performing hazard analysis, may therefore be expected.

Various government agencies may have the following involvement:

— ensuring that industry poses little threat to public safety from fire, explosion, or toxic emissions;
— ensuring that workers' safety is within acceptable limits, with regard largely to minor accidents and injury and chronic toxic effects;
— ensuring that public health is not affected adversely by chronic and acute toxic effects of industry;
— ensuring that damage to the environment (including people) in the form of dust, smoke, noise, odours, gas, and liquid pollutants is minimized;
— ensuring that land-use proposals (concerned with large areas rather than specific industries) involving hazardous industry zoning are appropriate;
— ensuring that emergency planning is appropriate for hazardous industry and surrounding areas.

Quantitative and qualitative hazard analysis

Technological hazards can be analysed and described either quantitatively or qualitatively.

Quantitative analysis (or "quantitative risk assessment") uses statistical, mathematical, and engineering concepts to arrive at the probability of a specific level of harm. For example, the probability of fatality caused by living within 500 metres of the industry may be described as 1×10^{-5} per year.

This form of analysis is useful for making decisions about the siting of hazardous industry, because it provides an estimate of the risk, which can be compared with risk criteria; this is called "risk assessment"). It requires the use of mathematical and statistical techniques, a knowledge of engineering, and familiarity with the particular type of industry. It is not necessary to perform a quantitative hazard analysis of an industry to develop emergency preparedness strategies for that industry and the surrounding community. However, those involved in emergency management should have some knowledge of quantitative hazard analysis if the scope and interpretation of such analyses are to be appropriate.

Qualitative analysis, using techniques such as those described in this chapter, will provide much useful information for emergency preparedness including:

— the types of hazard arising from the industrial activity;
— the nature of those hazards;
— the way in which those hazards may affect the community and the environment;
— the hazards that are the most serious, and should therefore be considered first and most urgently for emergency preparedness.

Because of the importance and widespread use of quantitative industrial hazard analysis, a general description of some of the methods is given below. An example of hazard description, using the qualitative hazard analysis techniques outlined earlier in this section, is also provided.

Quantitative industrial hazard analysis methods
Figure 17 shows a quantitative process often used in industrial hazard analysis.

Defining risk criteria
Risk criteria are defined for the industry's possible impact on workers and the community (6, 7). These criteria are the minimum acceptable risk levels, and may take five forms:

Fig. 17. **A quantitative industrial hazard analysis process**

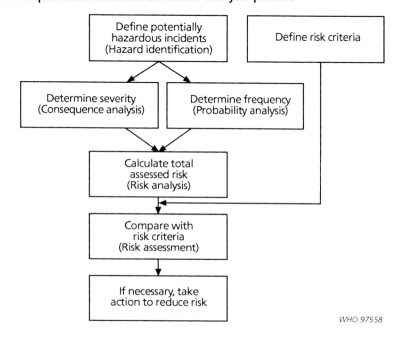

— individual fatality risk criteria;
— individual injury risk criteria;
— societal risk criteria;
— risk of property damage and accident propagation criteria;
— biophysical environment risk criteria.

Table 7 shows the individual fatality risk criteria and Table 8 the injury risk criteria accepted in many countries (7).

Societal risk criteria combine the probability of a hazardous event with the number of people killed. This takes into account the population density in the vicinity of a hazardous industry, and is otherwise known as an "F–N" curve, the cumulative frequency (F) of killing n or more people (N). No limits of acceptability for this criteria have been set in most countries and each case is judged by the individual risk levels and the population density.

Property damage and accident propagation criteria as well as injury risk criteria are based on heat radiation level and explosion overpressure. These criteria are intended to reduce risk to neighbouring structures and activities, particularly those of a hazardous nature, and to people, especially in residential areas. The criteria often used are shown in Table 9 (7).

The upper limit for heat radiation in industrial areas is that at which:

— there is a possibility of fatality from instantaneous exposure;
— there is spontaneous ignition of wood after long exposure;
— unprotected steel will reach thermal stress temperatures that can cause failure;
— pressure vessels need to be relieved to prevent failure.

The upper limit for explosion overpressure is that at which houses would be badly cracked and/or made uninhabitable.

Consideration should also be given to lower-risk events that might generate higher levels of heat radiation and explosion overpressure.

The biophysical environment risk criteria typically dictate that industrial developments should not be sited near sensitive natural environmental areas where:

Table 7. **Individual fatality risk criteria**

Land use or activity	Individual fatality risk per year
Hospitals, schools, child-care facilities, old-age housing	0.5×10^{-6}
Residential, hotels, motels, tourist resorts	1×10^{-6}
Commercial developments, including retail centres, offices, and entertainment centres	5×10^{-6}
Sporting complexes and recreation spaces	10×10^{-6}
Industrial	50×10^{-6}

Table 8. **Injury risk criteria**[a]

Cause of damage	Land use	Level	Probability per year
Heat radiation	Residential	4.7 kW/m^2	50×10^{-6}
Explosion overpressure	Residential	7 kPa	50×10^{-6}
Toxic concentrations	Residential	May cause serious injury	10×10^{-6}
		May cause irritation to eyes/throat, coughing, or other acute physiological responses	50×10^{-6}

[a] Reproduced from reference 7 by permission of NSW Department of Urban Affairs and Planning, Australia.

Table 9. **Property damage and accident propagation criteria**

Cause of damage	Land use	Level	Risk
Heat radiation	Residential	4.7 kW/m^2	50×10^{-6}
	Industrial	23 kW/m^2	50×10^{-6}
Explosion overpressure	Residential	7 kPa	50×10^{-6}
	Industrial	14 kPa	50×10^{-6}

— the effects of the more likely accidental emissions may threaten the long-term viability of the ecosystem or of any species within it;
— the probability of impacts that may threaten the long-term viability of the ecosystem or of any species within it is not substantially lower than the background level of threat to the ecosystem (7).

Again, these criteria need to be interpreted rather freely and applied on a case-by-case basis.

Defining potentially hazardous incidents

The types of incident usually examined by hazard analysis include:

— fire (including flash fire);
— vapour cloud explosion (confined or unconfined);
— boiling liquid/expanding vapour explosion (BLEVE);
— dust explosion and other types of explosion;
— toxic gas escapes;
— toxic fumes from fires.

Hazards to the biophysical environment, however, have been largely ignored in many studies.

Techniques for hazard identification include:

— past experience (limited to common and known hazards);
— engineering codes and standards (incomplete and generally limited to minor hazards);

- company and historical records (limited by the completeness of databases and to known hazards);
- checklists (limited because they are closed sets and may stifle more rigorous techniques);
- hazard index methods (e.g. Dow Chemical Company Fire and Explosion Index; Mond Fire, Explosion and Toxicity Index; Instantaneous Fractional Annual Loss (IFAL) technique; these methods are also used to determine severity and techniques for loss control);
- failure modes and effects analysis (FMEA);
- hazard and operability study (HAZOP);
- event and fault tree analysis (also used in severity and probability analysis).

FMEA and HAZOP are the recommended analytical techniques (8) and are supplemented by the others. HAZOP is briefly described below.

Hazard and operability study. The HAZOP is a form of hazard identification. It involves the study of flow–piping and instrumentation diagrams, section by section, by a team of engineers and technicians who participate in the plant design and will be involved in its operation. The study evaluates deviations from the normal operation of the plant, their consequences, and the efficacy of control systems. The following list of keywords may be used in a HAZOP.

- high flow
- low flow
- high level
- low level
- zero flow, empty
- reverse flow
- high pressure (venting, relief rate)
- low pressure (venting, relief rate)
- high temperature
- low temperature
- impurities (gaseous, liquid, solid)
- change in composition, change in concentration, 2-phase flow, reactions
- testing (equipment, product)

- plant items (operable, maintainable)
- electrical (area classification, isolation, earthing)
- instruments (sufficient for control, too many, correct location)
- toxicity
- services required (air, nitrogen, water, etc.)
- materials of construction (vessels, pipelines, pumps)
- commissioning
- start-up
- shutdown (isolation, purging)
- breakdown (power, failure, air, steam, water, vacuum, fuel, vents, computer, other)
- effluent (gaseous, liquid, solid)
- noise (sources, is it a problem, control measures)
- fire/explosion
- safety equipment (personal, fire detection, fire fighting, means of escape)
- quality and consistency
- output (reliability and bottlenecks)
- efficiency/losses
- simplicity.

Not all keywords apply to a particular section of a process or industry. The keywords, tailored for chemical processes, are intended as a checklist, but also as prompts for investigating possible process deviations. HAZOPs can be done only by those with sufficient experience and expertise to understand the plant processes thoroughly.

Determining severity

The method for determining the severity (assessing the effects) of an identified hazard depends on the type of incident, e.g. fire, vapour cloud explosion, BLEVE, dust, explosion, toxic gas escape, or toxic fumes from fires. The following is an example of a typical methodology for fires:

- Identify source, e.g. leak or spill of the product.
- Determine the nature of the fire, e.g. a jet flame around a leak or a pool fire.
- Assess the heat of combustion and amount of heat radiated.
- Assess whether the flame is likely to impinge on critical structures or areas.
- Compare heat radiation with tables of effects.
- Determine the need for, and best means of, protection.

The amount of heat radiated may be determined using the *point source method* or *view factor method*. The result from either method is an intensity in kilowatts per square metre (kW/m^2), which can be compared with the effects for different radiant heat levels in Table 10. A more detailed description of the effect of heat radiation on the human body is given in Table 11.

Thus, injury to people, or fatality, is dependent not only on the level (intensity) of radiant heat (in kW/m^2) but also on the duration of exposure. A further factor is the variation of the effects of heat on different people. The sensitivity of individuals in any given population to a harmful effect varies, and can be described using a mathematical model (e.g. probit function).

Severity determination for each type of event has its own techniques, methodologies, and assumptions. The end result of the severity determination step will be an assessment of the degree of damage or harm (often including probability statements regarding the degree of harm) from each identified event.

Table 10. **Effects of heat radiation**

Heat radiation level (kW/m^2)	Effect
1.2	Equivalent to heat from summer sun at noon
1.6	Minimum level at which pain can be felt
5	Will cause pain in 15–20 seconds and at least second-degree burns after 30 seconds
6	Probability of person being able to take cover is 50%
12.5	Heats wood to temperature where pilot ignition (e.g. spark) will start fire
13	Probability of person being able to take cover is effectively zero
25	Spontaneous ignition of wood. Thin insulated steel sections can reach a temperature at which thermal stresses cause failure
75	100% fatality — 5 seconds

Table 11. **Effects of heat radiation on humans**[a]

Heat radiation level (kW/m^2)	Approximate time (in seconds) to:		
	pain	1st-degree burns	2nd-degree burns
1.6	150	—	—
3.1	22	—	—
4.7	14	20	30
6.3	9	14	22
9.4	5	8	14
12.6	4	5	8

[a] Reproduced from reference 9 by permission of the publisher.

Determining frequency

The determination of the frequency of events is based on the frequency of causes and is often described using "fault trees". If two causes are required to produce an event, the probability of the event occurring is the product of the probability of the causes. If two causes can produce the same event independently, the probability of each is added. Note that a cause of an event may itself have a cause. In order to attach a probability to any event, the fault trees must be traced back to causes with probabilities that are known or can be estimated. The more complex fault trees will often have the same cause for one or more events, and Boolean algebra is then needed to reduce the chains of cause and effect to an equation.

Data on the probability of occurrence of various events that cause hazardous incidents are highly comprehensive for some processes but non-existent for others. Many companies have databases of these events, which are generally confidential. Where data are not available, educated guesses are made.

Random number simulation analysis (RNSA), also known as the Monte Carlo method, uses a fault tree or similar logical model, but assigns probabilities as ranges, rather than as specific values; this gives more realistic results.

Once the probability of an event has been determined, the probabilities of the various consequences of the event should be determined. "Event trees" are the usual tool for determining the consequence probability. A common method using event trees is the technique for human error rate prediction (THERP), which concentrates on operator error in process control.

Calculating total assessed risk

Calculating the total assessed risk consists of two parts: combining the probability of an event occurring and the probability of its various possible consequences (e.g. an event may have a probability of x, and the probability of fatality of an individual at a given distance may be y — thus the risk of fatality would be the product xy); and combining all the various risks associated with a particular plant or industry, expressed as risk contours, societal risk curves, and total risk of harmful explosion overpressure at given points, etc. The calculations involved in

VULNERABILITY ASSESSMENT

estimating the total risk of a particular industry are normally sufficiently complex and lengthy to require a computer. Their results are expressed in the same terms as risk criteria.

Comparison with risk criteria
The risk analysis results are compared with the risk criteria (risk assessment) to determine the types of actions required to reduce risk.

Limitations and accuracy of quantitative hazard analysis
The outputs of quantitative hazard analysis suggest a degree of accuracy and reliability that they do not have. Furthermore, no two hazard analyses will yield the same answers for a given industry. The reasons for this are many, and include the following.

- *Quality of data on event probability.* The causal events for hazardous incidents are assigned probabilities, based either on experience or on educated guesswork. In either case, these events and their probabilities are central to the probability of occurrence of the hazardous incident, and any inaccuracy in causal event probability can greatly influence the end result.
- *Assumption and conservatism.* At many stages in the calculations and logical techniques used, assumptions must be made as to prevailing or expected conditions. To correct for error in these assumptions, most hazard analysts will be conservative in their estimates. The degree of conservatism will greatly affect the end result.
- *Compounding of errors.* Any error in assumptions or original probabilities of causal events will be compounded in further calculations. Because the calculations tend to contain many steps, each with a known or unknown degree of probable error, and the end results of the calculations are generally combined to give overall risk levels, the final degree of probable error can be very large. For example, a calculated risk of fatality at a given place relative to a hazardous industry can be in error by as much as one or two orders of magnitude (i.e. differ by a factor of 10 or 100).

Qualitative industrial hazard analysis methods
A qualitative analysis will identify hazards, and describe the hazards, the community, and likely effects on people, property, or the environment. Intensity, frequency/likelihood, extent, time-frame, and manageability might be used as hazard descriptors in the analysis.

Intensity
Typically, industrial hazard analysis deals with three intensity aspects of technological hazards: explosion overpressure, heat radiation, and toxicity.

Heat radiation has already been described (see page 49). Explosion overpressure is the blast of compressed air that emanates from an explosion and is expressed in kilopascals (kPa). Toxicity is much more difficult to quantify, as most data are based on estimates of the effects on humans or experimental animals. A number of indicators for toxicity are used, including immediate danger to life and health (IDLH), 50% lethal dose (LD_{50}), and 100% lethal dose (LD_{100}). Toxicity of a substance is also dependent on the effects of a given dose of toxic material on a given individual. This variable effect is often described using a probit function.

Frequency or likelihood
In a qualitative hazard analysis, the frequency or likelihood of an event is described in words such as "highly likely", "likely", "possible", "unlikely", etc. These words may be related to time periods, for example, "highly likely" may be defined as likely to occur once in any given year, where "unlikely" may be defined as once in a lifetime.

Extent
The likely extent of an industrial hazard analysis is a function of consequence and distance, or risk (consequence × probability) and distance. It can be described in terms of distance from the industrial site or the likely affected area.

Time-frame
Time-frame refers to:

— the time of day, week, or year when an emergency is likely to occur;
— the length of warning time;
— the length of time for which the surrounding area may be hazardous;
— the duration of the emergency operation and community recovery.

Manageability
The manageability of an industrial hazard for emergency preparedness purposes indicates what can be done about the hazard in terms of planning, training, and education, and carrying out drills. Regarding prevention, manageability of industrial hazards can be described in terms of the following types of controls, often called the "hierarchy of control":

— elimination (process or material);
— replacement (process or material);
— reduction (quantity of material, pressure, temperature, etc.);
— engineering control (over process or material);
— separation from people, property, or environment;
— administrative control;
— emergency procedures;
— personal protection.

Other hazard descriptions
Further examples of ways of describing hazards are given in the tables on the modified Mercalli scale, Beaufort scale, tsunami scale, dangerous goods classes, etc. in Annex 2.

Hazard and risk mapping
Maps are among the best ways to present vulnerability assessment results. They provide a familiar spatial dimension, and the characteristics of a given hazard can be overlaid on other types of information, such as features of the environment and a community's relevant characteristics.

Table 12. **Types of map**

Map type	Information shown
Hazard map	Shows relevant hazard characteristics, including extent
Risk map	Similar to hazard map, but also shows probability of occurrence of a hazardous event
Vulnerability map	Shows distribution of the elements of the community that may be harmed or damaged

There is some confusion about the terminology associated with hazard maps, with different disciplines using different names for the various types of map. Table 12 shows some of the more common types and indicates the information that may be shown on them. The degree of complexity of these maps varies, as well as the degree of expertise and the time and resources needed to develop them.

The value and use of hazard, risk, and vulnerability maps may be influenced by a number of important factors such as scale (and detail), units of measurement, and sampling (of data). However, provided that these factors are taken into account, hazard mapping is a powerful tool in helping describe the nature of hazards.

Scale
The scale of a map is the proportion that the map bears to the geographical area shown. Small-scale maps show large areas with little detail, large-scale maps show smaller areas with greater detail. Small-scale hazard maps that cover a large area, such as a province or country, are valuable for prioritizing areas that may need further analysis or are likely to require emergency planning. They are therefore useful for developing policy and for making decisions on emergency management resourcing. Large-scale hazard maps are of value for detailed emergency management work.

Units of measurement
The units of measurement used on a hazard map should be practical for emergency management purposes. For example, an earthquake hazard map can show the probability of either peak ground acceleration, which is the amount of ground movement, or intensity, in terms of the modified Mercalli scale.

The modified Mercalli scale is more useful for emergency management becauseit indicates what people's reactions might be and the types of damage that may occur. Moreover, given most people's perception of risk and understanding of technical terminology, it is better to express results in a more accessible manner. The modified Mercalli scale is more concrete, and therefore more readily understood. It is also more useful than the Richter scale, since the latter measures the seismic energy released by an earthquake, not the earthquake's effects.

This highlights a general principle of vulnerability assessment, as well as of hazard and risk mapping: the results of a vulnerability assessment should be expressed in terms that are of greatest value to emergency management, and those terms should be concrete and understandable.

Sampling

Sampling refers to both the number of areas from which data have been collected and the period of time over which the data were collected for a given area.

The accuracy of hazard maps is clearly dependent on the extent of the sampling (in terms of area and time span) on which they are based. For example, accurate and scientific earthquake data, particularly for low-intensity earthquakes, have only been gathered during the latter half of the 20th century (although it is possible to infer sources and intensities of earlier earthquakes from historical documents). Since earthquakes of a damaging intensity are relatively infrequent, the analysis of past events and probability predictions of future events should be treated with an appropriate degree of scepticism. That is, areas that are shown on these maps to have a low probability of earthquake may, in fact, have a medium to high probability.

Describing the community

Why describe the community?

The purpose of vulnerability assessment is to describe the interaction between hazards, the community, and the environment in order to develop programmes and strategies for protecting the community and the environment. Without knowledge of the community and environment, it is impossible to describe their vulnerability.

The characteristics shown in Table 13 are among those that can be used to describe a community.

Demography

Demography is the study of the statistics of human populations. Of the large quantities of data often available on the population of any given community, only

Table 13. **Some community characteristics**

Demography	*Culture*	*Economy*	*Infrastructure*	*Environment*
Population and age distribution	Traditions	Trade	Communication networks	Landforms
Mobility	Ethnicity	Agriculture/ livestock	Transportation networks	Geology
Useful skills	Social values	Investments	Essential services	Waterways
Hazard awareness	Religion	Industries	Community assets	Climate
Vulnerable groups	Attitudes to hazards	Wealth	Government structures	Flora and fauna
Health level	Normal food types		Resource base	
Education level	Eating habits			
Sex distribution	Power structures			

some are relevant to emergency management. These concern the number of people in the area of study, their distribution across the area, and any concentrations of vulnerable groups. Such groups may be vulnerable because of age (young or old), mobility (availability of transport), or disabilities. However, most people — not just these easily defined groups — are vulnerable to emergencies to some extent.

The following indicators are important as regards the community's capacity for response and recovery:

- Health indicators, which determine how much resistance people can offer to the health effects of an emergency; for example:
  — infant mortality rate indicates the health service coverage;
  — vaccination coverage rate indicates the extent and effectiveness of preventive programmes;
  — disease pattern indicates potential outbreaks of new disease or worsening of existing disease after an emergency;
  — malnutrition rate indicates how quickly and for how long feeding programmes may be needed.
- Educational indicators, which determine how sophisticated the role of the community can be in participating in response activities and the level and type of public message that can be used; for example:
  — literacy rate, which is important for assessing the level of community participation and response that can be planned for;
  — female literacy rate, which is important for the success of health education and public preparedness.

The best way to obtain demographic data on a community is to contact the government organization responsible. Data may be available in printed form or as computer files.

Another aspect of vulnerability is the ability of the community to manage hazards. Those who have a realistic perception of the hazards around them and are aware of the measures necessary to manage those hazards are better able to cope with emergencies. Certain communities will have particular skills that are useful in emergency management. For example, a mining community would probably be better able to cope following storm damage or an earthquake than urban dwellers, owing to the available technical skills, and rural communities would be more resilient than urban communities because of their greater self-sufficiency in normal times.

Culture

A community's culture, including its traditions, ethnicity, and social values, is highly relevant to emergency management. Attitudes towards hazards and vulnerability will be strongly influenced by attitudes towards nature, technology, the causation of accidents and emergencies, and the value of mitigating or contingent actions. Some communities, for example, accept that lives will inevitably be lost in emergencies and may be unwilling to take preventive, preparatory, or response actions.

Economy

The economy of the community requires protection, and the more sensitive and vulnerable sections of the economy require careful consideration in emergency management. It is likely that an emergency that causes considerable structural and environmental damage would devastate the local tourism industry, for example. Investment may also suffer because potential or current investors would regard the risks in the area as too high. Industries and trade might also suffer if disruption to transport and communications were to restrict access to goods and markets. Thus, the wealth of a community may also determine its resilience or its likelihood of sustaining harm.

Infrastructure

The infrastructure (both physical and organizational) of a community is often highly vulnerable to hazards, particularly natural hazards. A vulnerability assessment should consider any possible damage to power generation and distribution systems, water supplies, communications systems, etc. These are often referred to as "lifelines", and relevant considerations include:

— effect of loss of services on the community;
— possible extent of the damage;
— alternative means of supplying the service;
— time required for repairs;
— cost of repairs.

It is also important to have a basic description of the government structure, and of service and community organizations, since they will provide the mechanism for emergency management programmes and strategies.

Any other characteristics of a community that are relevant to emergency management should also be considered.

Environment

The environment is an important determinant of settlement patterns and lifestyles of communities; it can be defined as the natural surroundings, including plants and animals, water, air, and soil. Damage to any of these elements may affect other elements of the environment. Many hazards can adversely affect the environment, including chronic (continuous and low-level) or acute (sudden and high-level) pollution by hazardous materials.

Paradoxically, while the environment nurtures the community it can also be the source of some of the greatest natural hazards. Describing the environment in a vulnerability assessment will often identify some hazards that have not yet been considered.

Community and environment mapping

As with hazards, detailed information about a community can be documented effectively with maps. This is particularly true when the characteristics that describe the community vary systematically over a geographical area. The community information that can be mapped includes:

VULNERABILITY ASSESSMENT

- Population density
- Particularly vulnerable groups — prisons, mental hospitals, orphanages, homes for the disabled, and new and unplanned settlements
- Potential emergency shelter sites
- Community preparedness focal points
- Emergency services — police, fire, ambulance, civil protection, and armed forces
- Residences of essential staff
- Proposed food distribution points
- Water and sanitation information
- Health centres
- Warehouses
- Utility networks and distribution points — electricity, gas, water
- Communication networks
- Essential businesses and factories
- Fuel storage points and distribution sources
- Transport systems and networks
- Road exit points from district
- Ongoing routine maintenance of roads and utilities

Description of effects and vulnerability
How are effects and vulnerability described?

The way in which vulnerability and the effects of hazards are described will depend on the scope of the vulnerability assessment. If a community is assessed, a standard set of parameters to describe the effects (e.g. extent and number of services disrupted, number of homeless persons) can be used. For a hospital, however, other parameters (e.g. effect of loss of service on the community, emergency medical demands on the hospital, effects on staff, and cost of and time required for repairs) would be useful. Table 14 shows some possible parameters for describing community vulnerability and the effects of hazards on a community.

These possible parameters should be discussed with the planning group and modified if necessary. Each hazard should then be examined in detail, parameter by parameter, to estimate the degree of loss in relation to each parameter in the community. The differential vulnerability of parts of the community in respect of these parameters can also be described, and the results of the entire examination should be documented immediately. The planning group should also realize that one emergency may provoke others. There is usually, in fact, a cascade effect, more and different emergencies following the original. These, too should be planned for. There are also specific needs that can be predicted for different types of emergencies (*12*). In addition:

- *Volcanic eruptions.* Possible needs (and secondary effects) are similar to those for earthquakes within the area directly affected by the eruption; there may be population displacements.
- *Tsunamis* (tidal waves caused by earthquakes). Possible needs are similar to those of tropical storms plus floods, with the added complication of contamination of wells and agricultural land by salt water.
- *Epidemics.* Needs usually include specific drugs, transport, surveillance, improvement of water supplies, personal hygiene and sanitation; reinforcement of health service management may also be required.

Table 14. **Descriptive parameters for the potential effects of hazards**[a]

Effects	Measure	Losses	
		Tangible	Intangible
Deaths	Number of people	Loss of economically active individuals, cost of retrieval and burial	Social and psychological effects on remaining community
Injuries	Number and injury severity	Medical treatment, temporary loss of economic activity by productive individuals, reduced ability of medical facilities in dealing with normal cases	Social and psychological pain and recovery
Social disruption	Number of displaced and homeless persons	Temporary housing, recovery work, economic production	Psychological, social contacts, cohesion, community morale
Disruption of normal services and infrastructure damage	Services disrupted, location, degree of damage, down-time	Inconvenience and harm to service users, replacement and repair costs	Concern over loss of services
Private property damage	Property type, degree of damage, and location	Replacement and repair costs	Cultural losses, decreased self-sufficiency
Disruption to economy	Number of working days lost, volume of production lost, amount of trade lost	Value of lost production	Opportunities, competitiveness, reputation, increased vulnerability
Environmental damage	Scale and severity	Clean-up costs, repair costs	Consequences of poorer environment, health risks, risk of future disaster, increased vulnerability

[a] Reproduced from reference 10 by permission of the publisher.

VULNERABILITY ASSESSMENT

Effects and vulnerability mapping

On vulnerability maps, those aspects of the community (and often of the environment) that are vulnerable or at risk are overlaid with hazard information. This allows an estimate of the degree of harm or loss that may occur. The simplest way to produce such a map is to use a transparent, removable overlay on a base map. Even if a preparedness programme lacks the time and financial resources for vulnerability maps, the concept of mapping can still be used as an analogy. In determining the likely effects of hazards it is worth considering how the community is spatially related to the hazard.

It is equally possible to map the vulnerable aspects of the environment. This can be useful in the following areas:

- *Fire*. Which areas contain forest resources that might be destroyed? Are there fauna and flora that would be severely affected?
- *Hazardous materials*. Are there fishing areas downstream of industrial outfalls that might be affected by acute spills? Are there breeding grounds for waterfowl or fish downstream?
- *Oil pollution*. Are there fauna and flora likely to be affected by oil spills or by the use of oil dispersants? Are there areas that are used for recreation and tourism that may be affected adversely?

Geographical information systems

Geographical information systems (GIS) will be widely used in the future for hazard and vulnerability mapping. They are computer programs that combine a relational database with spatial interpretation and output. A more technical definition is "A system for capturing, storing, checking, integrating, analyzing and displaying data about the Earth that is spatially referenced. It is normally taken to include a spatially referenced database and appropriate applications software." (*11*).

It is possible to enter a variety of types of data, and relate them through formulae, or overlap them in a graphic presentation, either on screen or as a printed map. Use of GIS is increasing for the everyday administration of communities, and existing systems and information can be used for emergency management purposes. GIS allow the rapid analysis of large quantities of related data and can also be used as a predictive tool. When applied to hazard and vulnerability information, GIS can be employed for all aspects of emergency management.

An example of the use of GIS in preparedness and response is in the recording and analysis of data on large stores of hazardous materials. Government organizations often collect data on these stores for the purposes of licensing and public safety. If the data are entered into a GIS, the following information can rapidly be displayed in graphic form:

— locations of the largest stores;
— distances to the nearest fire station;
— who owns a particular storage area and their after-hours contact details;
— what material is stored, where on the site, etc.

GIS can be combined with a gas- or smoke-modelling program to determine the possible concentrations of gas, fumes, or smoke following an accidental release of hazardous material or a fire. The shortest routes from a given fire station to a given store can be calculated and possible evacuation routes plotted. This information can be used both for emergency planning in relation to the storage of hazardous materials and in the response to accidents involving hazardous materials.

Hazard prioritization

Why prioritize hazards?

In any community, resources for the management of hazards, vulnerability, and emergencies are limited. With the best of intentions, the constraints of time and money preclude protecting people, property, and the environment from every hazard. Therefore, it is crucial to decide which hazards should be dealt with most urgently and which should be dealt with later or not at all.

How to prioritize hazards

Determining which hazards to target for management is called "hazard prioritization", or "hazard ranking". There are a number of ways to prioritize hazards, two of which are discussed in the following paragraphs.

The key to prioritizing hazards is community involvement. As in the other steps of vulnerability assessment, consultative and participative processes are necessary. The commitment of those required to take action and those who may be affected by hazards is essential. Without it, the best emergency management strategies, based on the best of vulnerability assessments, may fail. Hence, the first step is to involve the relevant people.

Another reason for using consultative and participative processes in hazard prioritization is that the choices that need to be made to reduce the likely effects of hazards are political decisions. Some hazard mitigation and response strategies will only protect some people and others may not address the needs of the most vulnerable. The decisions as to who and what should be protected, and to what degree, should be made by the whole community.

The second step is to determine which criteria to use to rank the hazards. Criteria may include factors such as the probability of an emergency, the level of vulnerability of people or property or both, the degree of manageability, and whether the hazard may worsen and how quickly. There are a number of methods that use such criteria, including the FEMA (the United States Federal Emergency Management Agency) model and the SMUG ("seriousness", "manageability", "urgency", and "growth" — developed by the Tasmania State Emergency Service) hazard priority system, which are described below.

A simpler method has already been described in the section on hazard identification — the group technique for identifying hazards. Using this technique and a few simple criteria such as "risk" (the likelihood of a given level of harm), "manageability" (whether anything can be done about this hazard), and

VULNERABILITY ASSESSMENT

"vulnerability" (how damaging is the potential harm caused by this hazard), it is possible to rank community hazards. Community vulnerabilities can also be ranked in this way.

In prioritizing hazards there is no "right" answer, and there will be a number of hazards that are considered to be more serious than others. It may also be difficult to equate or compare different hazard analysis results. This is to be expected, since different hazards may have very different effects, and it is not always possible to compare hazards precisely. In short, resources should be committed to hazards that the community considers to be most serious, using whatever criteria of "seriousness" they deem correct. Hazard prioritization should be used as a guide to decision-making and modified to suit the requirements of particular communities.

The FEMA model

The FEMA model uses four criteria in an evaluation and scoring system — history, vulnerability, maximum threat, and probability (*12*):

- *History.* If a certain type of emergency has occurred in the past, it is known that there were sufficient hazardous conditions and vulnerability to cause the event. Unless these conditions no longer exist, or have been substantially reduced, a similar emergency may occur again. Lack of a past occurrence, however, does not mean that there is no future emergency potential.
- *Vulnerability.* This attempts to determine the number of people and the value of property that may be vulnerable, based on such factors as vulnerable groups (aged, disabled, and children); population densities; location of population groups; location and value of property; and location of vital facilities, e.g. hospitals. Overlaying hazard maps on a map of the community assists in this process.
- *Maximum threat.* This is essentially the worst case scenario; that is, it assumes the most serious event possible and the greatest impact. It is expressed in terms of human casualties and property loss. Secondary events (such as dam failure following an earthquake) also need to be considered.
- *Probability.* Probability is the likelihood of an event occurring, expressed in terms of chances per year that an event of a specific intensity (or greater) will occur. There is some link between probability and history; however, since some hazards are without historical precedent, an analysis of both history and probability is necessary.

An evaluation of low, medium, or high is made for each criterion shown in Table 15.

For each evaluation, score the following:

Low	1 point
Medium	5 points
High	10 points

Some criteria have been determined as more important than others, and the following weightings have been established:

History	×2
Vulnerability	×5
Maximum threat	×10
Probability	×7

A composite score for each hazard is arrived at by multiplying the score by the weighting, then adding the four results. Table 16 gives an example:

The FEMA model suggests a threshold of 100 points. All hazards that total more than 100 points may receive higher priority in emergency preparedness. Hazards totalling less than 100 points, while receiving a lower priority, should still be considered.

This process should be repeated for all identified hazards and for a range of scenarios with the same hazard.

Table 15. **The FEMA evaluation and scoring system**[a]

Criteria		Evaluation
History: whether an emergency event has occurred:	<2 times in 100 years	Low
	2–3 times in 100 years	Medium
	>3 times in 100 years	High
Vulnerability: of people	1%	Low
	1–10%	Medium
	>10%	High
of property	1%	Low
	1–10%	Medium
	>10%	High
Maximum threat: area of the community affected	5%	Low
	5–25%	Medium
	>25%	High
Probability: chances per year of an emergency	<1 in 1 000	Low
	1 in 1 000–1 in 10	Medium
	>1 in 10	High

[a] Reproduced from reference *12* by permission of the publisher, Emergency Management Australia (formerly Natural Disasters Organisation).

Table 16. **Sample use of the FEMA evaluation and scoring system**

Criteria	Evaluation	Score × weighting	Total
History	High	10 × 2	20
Vulnerability	Medium	5 × 5	25
Maximum threat	High	10 × 10	100
Probability	Medium	5 × 7	35
Total			*180*

VULNERABILITY ASSESSMENT

SMUG hazard priority system

The SMUG hazard priority system allows a direct comparison of a number of possible hazards, through ratings of high, medium, or low, against four separate criteria common to all hazards (*12*):

- *Seriousness.* The relative impact of a hazard, in terms of financial cost or number of people affected or both. If a hazard represents a threat to the greatest number of people or would cost the most (or both), that hazard is given a "high" rating. All identified hazards are rated as "high", "medium", or "low", in terms of seriousness. If the group cannot agree, the highest rating should be given.
- *Manageability.* "Can anything be done about the hazard?". If the impact of the hazard can be lessened, the rating for manageability would be "high". If it were manageable only after it had occurred, the rating would be "low".
- *Urgency.* "High" means that something should be done now, "medium" means something should be done in the near future, and "low" means there is no urgency and action can be deferred.
- *Growth.* If nothing is done about the hazard, will it grow worse or remain as it is? If the hazard would increase quickly, it is rated "high", if it would grow gradually, "medium", and if it would stay static, "low".

Once a relative rating has been allocated to all identified hazards according to these criteria, the list of hazards should be reviewed. Those with the most "high" ratings are the ones that warrant priority attention. It is very important to provide clear evidence to support the ratings. Table 17, for example, would be useful for recording decisions.

Example of use of prioritization techniques

There is a basic difference between the FEMA and SMUG hazard priority systems. In the FEMA model, each hazard is rated individually, using a number of quantitative criteria such as history and probability, and individually given a numerical score, based on the value of each of those criteria. The SMUG system, on the other hand, compares hazards directly using a number of criteria, in a stepwise fashion, and is qualitative.

Table 17. **The SMUG hazard priority system**[a]

Hazard	*Criteria*			
	Seriousness	*Manageability*	*Urgency*	*Growth*
Hazard A	H/M/L	H/M/L	H/M/L	H/M/L
Hazard B	H/M/L	H/M/L	H/M/L	H/M/L
Hazard C	H/M/L	H/M/L	H/M/L	H/M/L

[a] Reproduced from reference *12* by permission of the publisher, Emergency Management Australia (formerly Natural Disasters Organisation).

The FEMA model, because it judges each hazard individually in a numerical manner, may provide more satisfying results than the SMUG system if there are sound numerical data on the hazards in question. The SMUG system, on the other hand, allows close comparison of each hazard with the others on the basis of the given criteria and therefore allows a closer examination of the differences between hazards in a more holistic sense.

In the following example of prioritization, the possible effects of hazards that exist in and near a fictitious country town are summarized.

Example

The town is situated near a river and bordered on one side by a forest. It has a population of approximately 1200 people, evenly spread throughout the town. Most families have vehicles, there are no care homes for the elderly, and there is one school. The townspeople all speak the same language, have a similar cultural and ethnic background, and consider themselves self-sufficient in most respects. The town's economy is based on providing services to the surrounding rural community and there are also a few light industries. There is a strong feeling of pride in the town, and there are a number of active community groups. The town is the seat of local government for the area, but the services the local government provides mostly relate to road maintenance, garbage collection, and sewage disposal. The local government has not developed any emergency management strategies.

The river floods regularly, and major flooding has occurred about once every 40 years for the past century. Alterations to the environment upstream suggest that flooding may be more extreme in the future. Major floods have the potential to destroy the sewage treatment plant and contaminate water supplies, incapacitate all telephone and electricity services, destroy most bridges in the area, and cover many roads, forcing the evacuation of about 15% of all homes and disrupting half the town's light industries. It is not thought likely that many residents would be killed by floods while in their homes or during evacuation, but it is possible that some may be killed using flooded roads. A major flood has not occurred for many years and most residents do not perceive flood as a serious hazard.

The forest adjacent to the town is fairly dense and subject to selective logging. There have been frequent forest fires, some of which have threatened houses on the forest side of the town. The vegetation in the fields surrounding the town is generally kept low by grazing animals, but there are periods in summer following heavy rains when there is considerable growth of grass, which then dries. There is an active fire service in the town, but it is called only infrequently to fires. Telephone and electricity services may be disrupted by a severe fire and about 5% of houses may be burnt, but deaths and injuries are likely only among firefighters and during evacuation in the event of a serious fire. Geologists believe the area to be potentially subject to earthquakes, with a 10% chance of exceeding modified Mercalli VII intensity in a given 50-year period. The area has experienced one severe earthquake in known history, but this occurred before the town's construction, when the first settlers had only just arrived. Half of the town is built on alluvial soils that may be prone to liquefaction. Most buildings are of medium-quality masonry and timber construction, so that there is not much likelihood of building destruction or of a large number of deaths. The greatest risk is the destruction of all electricity, telephone, water supply, and sewage services, partial destruction of most bridges and many roads, and long-term disruption to light industry. There is no local knowledge of any earthquake hazard.

The town is almost totally dependent on the economic success of the surrounding rural areas — the raising of livestock for domestic consumption, for live export, and for export as meat products. There is a rudimentary quarantine system in place for the entire country, but no planning for response to an outbreak of exotic disease among livestock. An uncontrolled outbreak of such a disease would lead to the quarantining of the entire country and an immediate end to all animal product exports. This would cause an almost immediate closure of most businesses in the town, resulting in widespread bankruptcy and unemployment. It is highly unlikely that the disease would be a direct cause of human deaths or injuries. Local farmers and veterinarians are aware of the possibility of exotic animal disease, but unaware of the possible implications of an uncontrolled outbreak.

Using the SMUG hazard priority system

How would the SMUG system prioritize the four hazards of flood, forest fire, earthquake, and exotic animal disease for this town, based on the information given in the example? Table 18 shows a possible prioritization.

To summarize the SMUG prioritization, the hazards should be ranked in the order shown in Table 19.

Using the FEMA model

Using the FEMA model to prioritize the hazards described in the example produces the results summarized in Table 20.

To complete this FEMA prioritization, a number of assumptions have been made about the frequency and consequences of an event; in a real analysis these assumptions would have to be explicitly written down. According to the principles of the FEMA model, where a score in excess of 100 suggests that management of that hazard is required, the earthquake hazard would not be considered particularly serious compared with the other three.

Comparing FEMA and SMUG results

Table 21 compares the FEMA rating with the SMUG rating for the hazards described in the example.

The two prioritization systems may, in reality, provide different rankings because they use very different criteria, and some variation between their results would be

Table 18. Sample use of SMUG hazard priority system

Hazard	Criteria							
	Seriousness		Manageability		Urgency		Growth	
Flood	May cause some deaths, will cause considerable inconvenience and property and services damage	H	Manageable in that future developments can be protected from flood damage and response plans can be developed	H	As major floods occur infrequently, may not be considered too urgent by some	M	This problem will become significantly worse if there is no control of development in the flood plain	M
Forest fire	May cause some deaths, some property and services damage	M	Hazard reduction and fire breaks may completely eliminate the threat	H	Moderately urgent, but will be more urgent during dry season	M	If hazard reduction measures are not undertaken this hazard may become worse	L
Earthquake	Will destroy services, therefore economic and social costs will be high	M	May not be cost-effective to mitigate effects by structural means; response and recovery plans would alleviate effects	L	Currently impossible to predict, but probably an infrequent occurrence; overall impact over the years is low	L	Will not become a greater problem if not addressed now	L
Exotic animal disease	Will cause extreme social and economic disruption; many effects may be irreversible	H	Can be managed with good quarantine procedures and effective response procedures	H	Because of serious consequences should be addressed as soon as possible	H	Will not become a greater problem if not addressed now	L

VULNERABILITY ASSESSMENT

Table 19. **Sample hazard rating**

Hazard	SMUG prioritization
Flood	2
Forest fire	3
Earthquake	4
Exotic animal disease	1

Table 20. **Sample use of the FEMA model**

Criteria	Flood	Forest fire	Earthquake	Exotic animal disease
History	(medium) $5 \times 2 = 10$	(high) $10 \times 2 = 20$	(low) $1 \times 2 = 2$	(low) $1 \times 2 = 2$
Vulnerability	(high) $10 \times 5 = 50$	(medium) $5 \times 5 = 25$	(medium) $5 \times 5 = 25$	(high) $10 \times 5 = 50$
Maximum threat	(medium) $5 \times 10 = 50$	(low) $1 \times 10 = 10$	(medium) $5 \times 10 = 50$	(high) $10 \times 10 = 100$
Probability	(medium) $5 \times 7 = 35$	(high) $10 \times 7 = 70$	(low) $1 \times 7 = 7$	(medium) $5 \times 7 = 35$
Total	145	125	84	187

Table 21. **Comparison of hazard ratings**

Hazard	SMUG prioritization	FEMA prioritization
Flood	2	2
Forest fire	3	3
Earthquake	4	4
Exotic animal disease	1	1

expected. Experience has shown, however, that they tend to produce similar results.

It therefore seems that exotic animal disease is the greatest hazard for the town in the example, with flood coming second. Most of the hazards for this town are relatively minor since there is little expectation of loss of human life, but there are some significant economic implications.

Recommending action

At the end of a vulnerability assessment there should be conclusions, recommendations, and a summary.

The conclusions are a logical extension of previous work and focus on work already performed. They are based on the information in the vulnerability assessment and should not introduce any new facts. Recommendations focus on the work that needs to be accomplished in emergency preparedness, response, and recovery. The summary is a short synopsis of the entire work, containing the method, planning group composition, very brief conclusions, and a list of the recommendations.

There are three important questions that the planning group should consider when writing the conclusions and recommendations:

- To whom is the planning group to report the conclusions and recommendations of the vulnerability assessment?

  Reporting will normally be to the individual or organization that authorized the vulnerability assessment.

- How does the planning group gain support for the conclusions and recommendations?

  To gain the support of the authorizing individual or organization, a copy of the vulnerability assessment should be provided and a summary of the assessment should be given in an oral presentation.

- What form should the conclusions and recommendations take?

  The conclusions should be a series of short statements of fact and/or interpretations of information. Justification and supporting arguments for these conclusions should be contained in the body of the vulnerability assessment with cross-references to specific sections of the assessment if necessary. The recommendations for action that could or should be taken are based on the conclusions; they provide the link to the rest of the emergency preparedness process.

Summary

- Vulnerability assessment is a procedure for identifying hazards, describing community vulnerability, and determining the effects of potential emergencies on communities.
- Communities, hazards, and the environment interact with each other.
- A vulnerability assessment should be developed using a rational process.
- A planning group and community consultation are essential for the efficient development of an appropriate vulnerability assessment.
- Different people think of hazards, risk, and vulnerability in different ways, and this perception will affect their actions.
- A description of the effects of hazards and potential emergencies on communities must form the basis of emergency preparedness.

References

1. Plough A, Krimsky S. The emergence of risk communication studies: social and political context. *Science, technology and human values*, 1987, 12(3–4):4–10.

2. British Medical Association. *The Cambridge University Casualty Database — living with risk.* London, Wiley, 1987.

3. Slovic P, Fischoff B, Lichtenstein S. Characterising perceived risk. In: Kates RW et al., eds. *Perilous progress: technology as hazard.* Boulder, CO, Westview, 1985.

VULNERABILITY ASSESSMENT

4. Smith DI. Damage estimation and preparedness for dam failure flooding. *ANCOLD bulletin*, 1992, 90:26.

5. *Australian rainfall and runoff — a guide to flood estimation*. Canberra, The Institution of Engineers, 1987.

6. *Risk criteria for land-use planning in the vicinity of major industrial hazards*. London, Health and Safety Executive, 1989.

7. *Risk criteria for land use safety planning*. Sydney, Department of Planning, 1990 (Hazardous Industry Advisory Paper No. 4).

8. Slater D, Corran E, Pitblado RM. *Major industrial hazards — project report*. Sydney, The Warren Centre, University of Sydney, 1986.

9. *Risk analysis methodology. Procedure for estimating the consequences of releases of hazardous substances*. Melbourne, ICI Australia, 1989 (Process Safety Guide No. 10, Part II).

10. *An overview of disaster management*. Geneva, United Nations Disaster Relief Organization, 1992.

11. Dale PF, McLaughlin JD. *Land information management: an introduction with special reference to cadastral problems in Third World countries*. Oxford, Clarendon, 1988.

12. *Australian emergency manual: community emergency planning guide*, 2nd ed. Canberra, Natural Disasters Organisation, 1992.

Chapter 4
Emergency planning

Introduction
What is an emergency plan?
An emergency plan is an agreed set of arrangements for responding to and recovering from emergencies; it describes responsibilities, management structures, strategies, and resources.

Why develop plans?
People who do not believe planning is necessary argue that:

— everybody knows what to do;
— emergencies are unpredictable and impossible to plan for;
— people do not follow plans in emergencies;
— developing emergency plans will worry the public.

These arguments are considered in the following paragraphs.

Everybody knows what to do
In a well prepared community or organization, all those involved in emergency management may be aware of their role, but that role may not have been considered in the overall context of what needs to be done. It is possible that the roles of some people may conflict with those of others.

Have all the tasks required for effective, efficient, and appropriate emergency response and recovery strategies been allocated? Without emergency planning, it is probable that many fundamental and necessary responsibilities will not have been allocated, and this may be realized only during or after the emergency event. While people may know their own role, they may be unaware of the responsibilities of others with whom they must interact. Without emergency planning and appropriate training, it is unlikely that people will understand how they should work with others.

Have all the management functions been decided and the potential problems solved? Without emergency planning, confusion will arise over management arrangements during an emergency and this may result in minor crises.

How are people newly appointed to a job going to be informed of their emergency management role? A written plan is the best way to begin their education.

Emergencies are unpredictable and planning for them is impossible
It is precisely because emergencies are difficult to predict and the effects are uncertain that vulnerability assessments are performed and emergency plans developed.

"The aim is to reduce uncertainty through anticipation of what the situation requires ... planning is not a cure-all. All emergencies present in some measure unanticipated contingencies and difficulties. In those cases, action has to become innovative and emergent. However, planning will clearly improve any organized response effort by identifying what in all probability must be done, how it should be done, and what resources will be needed. In this manner, organized response can be made more highly predictable and efficient." (1)

People do not follow plans in emergencies

It is common for people not to refer to written emergency plans during the more critical moments of emergencies. However, if they have a basic understanding of the content and intent of a well prepared emergency plan, their actions are more likely to be appropriate. It is not just the written plan that is important — the planning process itself is important because it is a tool for problem-solving and education.

The development of emergency plans will unduly worry the public

The arousal of public anxiety is a common political objection to emergency planning. However, if there is a realistic threat to life and the environment, something must be done about it. The planning process is designed to achieve this end.

What can emergency plans do?

Emergency planning is about protecting life, property, and the environment. Evidence proves that planning increases this protection. Figure 18 illustrates one aspect of the value of emergency planning, that of effective warnings. The horizontal scale indicates the number of people at risk from a dam failure; the vertical scale indicates the number of actual deaths from recorded dam failures. The two curves on the graph represent the number of deaths due to dam failure for a given size of the population, with and without sufficient warning. The data for this graph come from actual events. The warnings were the result of emergency planning, and the graph clearly demonstrates that emergency planning reduces harm to people.

Fig. 18. **Deaths due to dam failure and extreme flood events — with and without warning systems**[a]

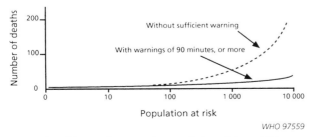

[a] Reproduced from reference 2 by permission of the publisher.

Fig. 19. **Context of emergency plans for a community**

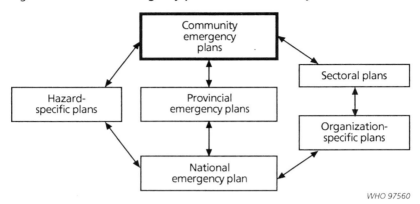

Context of emergency plans

Emergency plans do not operate in a vacuum — they are linked to the culture and perception of risk of those developing the plans and of those for whom the plans are developed. They must be developed to suit the context in which they will operate, which is one of the reasons that adapting an existing plan to a different area does not work. Quite apart from their application to general emergency management, community emergency plans should be considered in the context of other emergency plans — plans at other administrative levels, those that operate at the same level, and any plans developed for specific hazards or by other organizations (see Fig. 19).

Community, provincial, and national emergency plans are multisectoral. They include communications, search and rescue, police and security, health, social welfare, and transport and lifelines sectors, and coordinate the emergency work at each administrative level. Sectoral plans (sometimes called "functional plans") describe the management, resources, and strategies within one of these six sectors. Organization-specific plans are useful for members of a given organization, whether public or private, military, or nongovernmental. They describe in detail how that organization will fulfil its assigned roles and responsibilities. Hazard-specific plans may be developed for hazards such as flood, hazardous materials incidents, and epidemics.

Some principles of emergency planning

Emergency planning is based on certain principles (*1*) in order to facilitate decision-making. Planning:

— is a continuous process;
— attempts to reduce the unknowns in an emergency;
— aims to evoke appropriate actions;
— should be based on what is likely to happen;
— must be based on knowledge;
— should focus on principles;

- is partly an educational activity;
- always has to overcome resistance;
- should be simple enough to avoid confusion;
- should be flexible enough to adapt to any situation;
- can only define the starting point for response and recovery operations;
- should allow for the development of emergent strategies.

The prerequisites for planning are:
- recognition that hazards and vulnerability exist and that emergencies can occur;
- awareness among the community, government, and decision-makers of the need to plan and of the benefits of planning;
- appropriate legislation to guarantee implementation of the plan;
- a designated organization responsible for coordinating both planning and response and recovery in the event of an emergency.

The planning process will produce:
- an understanding of organizational roles in response and recovery;
- a strengthening of emergency management networks;
- improved community awareness and participation;
- effective response and recovery strategies and systems;
- a simple and flexible written plan.

The written plan itself is only one outcome of the planning process. Emergency planning does not require the creation of a new emergency management organization; it should make use of the abilities and resources of existing organizations.

An emergency planning process

The *process* of emergency planning is of major importance: if this process is not rational and appropriate, it is unlikely that the plans produced will be of value.

The planning process described here is a series of rational steps for producing an emergency plan; each of these steps involves standard management methods. This process can be applied to any community, organization, or activity, e.g. the health sector in general, hospitals, and search and rescue organizations. It is intended primarily for preparedness, but can be used equally well for planning during response and recovery operations.

Each step of the planning process is defined briefly here (see Fig. 20), and discussed in greater detail later in the chapter. These steps must be documented, and the written emergency plan will consist of the results of each step.

- *Project definition* determines the aim, objectives, scope, and context of an emergency plan, describes the tasks required and the resources needed to perform these tasks (see Chapter 1 and Annex 1). Recommendations based on the vulnerability assessment should be used in the planning process.
- A representative *planning group* is essential for emergency planning. Without such a group it will be difficult to gather the required information and

Fig. 20. **An emergency planning process**

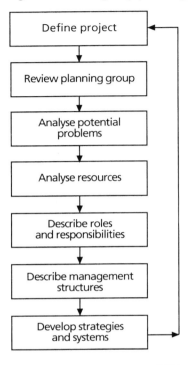

WHO 97561

gain the commitment of key people and organizations. There may be a need to review any existing planning group to assess its appropriateness. The composition of the planning group may change during the planning process.
- *Analysis of potential problems* examines in more detail the hazards and vulnerabilities, their causes, possible preventive strategies, response and recovery strategies, and trigger events for these strategies. It will provide information for later steps of the process.
- The *resource analysis* asks what resources are required, what is available, what is the variation between requirement and availability, and who is responsible.
- A description of *roles and responsibilities* outlines who does what.
- The *management structure* involves the command of individual organizations and control across organizations.
- Development of *strategies and systems* is concerned with response and recovery strategies and the systems that will support them.

Some planning groups may choose to alter the sequence of these steps, perhaps analysing resources before potential problems, or describing the management structure before describing roles and responsibilities.

Planning group review

A planning group is essential to developing appropriate emergency plans.

> "Well-prepared (emergency) plans specify what will be done, where, when, and by whom, to meet the specific demands of emergency conditions. Such plans can be developed only by representatives of operating departments and non-government groups with emergency missions. Paper plans prepared by the emergency program manager working alone, with little participation by operating departments, are of little value. In an actual emergency they will not be used. The development of a written plan, therefore, is not an end in itself. A written emergency plan does not guarantee that actual operations will be effective. But the process of planning that leads to the development of a written plan is extremely valuable. This is because the officials who are responsible for emergency operations have spent time determining which official will do what and how operations will be coordinated." (3)

Some criteria for selecting members of a planning group follow. These people should be:

— aware of the emergency management roles of their organization;
— actively involved in preparedness, responses, or recovery;
— of sufficient seniority to commit their organization to planning group decisions;
— capable of contributing to the planning group's work.

These criteria represent desirable attributes, but it is unlikely that every planning group member will fulfil them. The planning group should be small enough to be functional, and will generally include only one representative from each organization. The appropriateness of members of an *existing* planning group can be assessed in the same way.

Potential problem analysis

Introduction

The planning group should be briefed on the results of the vulnerability assessment, consider the recommendations of this assessment, and begin planning.

Potential problem analysis (4) is a technique for identifying preventive strategies and response and recovery strategies for problems that could arise in a given situation. Its value is that it systematically breaks down a problem into its components. Applied to emergency management, it can lead to innovative and effective strategies. The technique involves:

— identifying a hazard or hazardous situation;
— listing potential problems;
— determining causes;
— developing preventive strategies;
— developing response and recovery strategies, and trigger events for these strategies.

Preventive strategies are ways of reducing the probability of the problem, thereby reducing susceptibility. Response and recovery strategies are ways of reducing the seriousness of a problem that does occur, thereby increasing resilience.

At least two things are required to initiate a response or recovery strategy: a trigger event, and a person or organization responsible for initiating the strategy. The trigger event should indicate when the strategy is required; it could be an alarm, a warning, or the emergency itself. The responsible person or organization should be capable of initiating the strategy and the responsibility should be predetermined. To take a simple example, when flood water (hazard) reaches the 2-metre level at a particular bridge (trigger), a landowner (responsible person) contacts three neighbours so that they can move their animal stock to higher ground (response strategy).

A potential problem analysis can be performed by one person alone, but much better results will be obtained by a planning group. The planning group will also have a greater commitment to the strategies if it has been involved in their development.

How to perform a potential problem analysis

Consider a fire in a multistorey hospital as an example for a potential problem analysis. A vulnerability assessment on this hospital would reveal many of the potential problems that can be explored. Those that may be identified by a planning group might include:

— smoke, causing visibility problems;
— toxic smoke and fumes, causing lung damage to occupants;
— people trapped by smoke and flames;
— death due to smoke and flames;
— fire damage to property;
— water damage to equipment from sprinkler systems;
— threat of fire to adjacent buildings.

The results of a potential problem analysis can be recorded in tabular form (see Table 22).

Table 22. **Sample potential problem analysis**[a]

Hazard: ....

Potential problem	Cause	Preventive strategies	Response and recovery strategies	Trigger events
_____	_____	_____	_____	_____
_____	_____	_____	_____	_____
_____	_____	_____	_____	_____
_____	_____	_____	_____	_____

[a] Reproduced from reference 4 by permission from Kepner-Tregoe Inc., Princeton, NJ, USA. All rights reserved.

The next step is to consider causes in order to develop appropriate and effective preventive strategies and response and recovery strategies. The example can be extended with the potential problems relating to smoke. Some sources of smoke problems include:

- smoke caused by the ignition of garbage or other material that should have been removed;
- toxic smoke caused by burning of synthetic materials in furnishings;
- smoke caused by continued supply of oxygen to fire;
- smoke and fumes caused by applying an extinguishing agent inappropriate for the type of fire.

Listed below are some examples of preventive strategies for the smoke problem:

- reduce quantity of synthetic furnishings in the building (usually not cost-effective but worth considering);
- ensure appropriate housekeeping to reduce the amount of combustible material available (material that is not for immediate use in a given room should be stored in dedicated areas; garbage should be removed regularly);
- develop systems for reducing air flow to a fire (e.g. automatic or manual shut-off of air conditioning, closing of doors and windows);
- educate building occupants about the dangers of smoke and the best means to avoid it (e.g. staying close to the floor when leaving a building);
- train building occupants in the use of fire extinguishers.

Some possible response and recovery strategies include:

- shut off air conditioning as soon as fire is discovered (this may reduce the amount of oxygen that reaches the fire and the smoke produced);
- close all doors and windows;
- leave building in an organized manner;
- use fire extinguishers that are appropriate for the type of fire.

The trigger event and responsible person for setting in motion the response and recovery strategies must be determined by the planning group and documented.

Each of the other potential problems should then be considered in turn.

The technique of potential problem analysis is a powerful tool for developing emergency management strategies. It will produce the best results when used by a planning group because input comes from people with a variety of backgrounds and points of view. Members of the group will also inspire each other to develop new ideas. Equally important, since the group will be responsible for implementing the preventive and response and recovery strategies, is that group members should be involved in and committed to developing the strategies.

An interesting feature of potential problem analysis is that the same set of strategies for different potential problems will keep recurring. This is to be expected. The number of strategies for dealing with any complex set of problems is finite and many of them will be applicable to quite different problems.

Table 23. **Using the outputs of a potential problem analysis**

Output	Use
Possible preventive strategies	Add to existing prevention programmes
Possible response and recovery strategies	Determine whether existing resources will support a particular strategy Ensure that responsibilities for strategies have been assigned Develop further strategies for use in response and recovery
Trigger events	Ensure that trigger events are part of the alerting and warning system

Using the outputs of a potential problem analysis

The outputs of a potential problem analysis can be used in various ways (see Table 23), most of which are later steps in the planning process.

Resource analysis

Introduction

The vulnerability assessment describes the vulnerability of a community and the effects of hazards and recommends certain actions. The potential problem analysis suggests some response and recovery strategies. It is now necessary to determine what resources can be applied.

A "resource", as the term is used in this manual, is anything of value or use in emergency management, including people, training, equipment, facilities, materials, and money.

Why analyse emergency management resources?

There are a number of reasons for analysing emergency management resources. One is to ensure that possible preparedness, response, and recovery strategies can be supported by the appropriate resouces. Another is to ensure that preparedness is coordinated. There are many possible preparedness strategies, and a number of organizations will potentially be involved. The act of analysing resources will provide these organizations with shared information and goals, and will lead to greater coordination without which many organizations may well be poorly or inappropriately prepared. It is also crucial to know which resources are available for use in emergencies and who is responsible for supplying them.

How to perform a resource analysis

In a resource analysis, the following questions are asked (in the order given):

- What are the possible or proposed strategies?
- What resources are required?
- What resources are available?
- Who is responsible for these resources?
- What is the difference between the requirements and availability?
- If there is a shortfall, who is responsible for correcting it?
- Is the use of the resources in this area cost-effective?

Resource requirements should be identified for preparedness, response, and recovery. The potential problem analysis will have suggested some strategies, and these should be listed along with resources necessary to support them. If the planning group can think of any more strategies that may be required they should write them down. A five-column table can be constructed using the following headings: Strategies, Resources required, Resources available, Difference, and Responsible organization. At this stage it is best not to reject suggested resources, but to write them down uncritically.

When some *required* resources have been listed, *available* resources should be identified. The expertise and knowledge of the planning group are invaluable in determining what is available.

The third part of the resource analysis is to determine the difference between what is required and what is available. If the resource is available or in place, responsibility for providing it should be noted. If the resource is not available, the following further questions should be asked:

- Who should be responsible for providing this resource?
- Will it have a significant effect on the hazard or vulnerability?
- Will it be cost-effective?

If resources are available that are not required, the following questions may be asked:

- Has the resource requirement been poorly described?
- Are time and money being spent on resources that are not required?
- How can the time and money be used better?

It may be worthwhile to discuss the benefit of possible additional resources and weigh this against the cost. Resource-sharing with other organizations or communities may be considered. If a decision is made to acquire additional resources, it should be justified in a rational way. Similarly, a decision to shed apparently unnecessary resources should also be justified.

Resources for emergency preparedness, response, and recovery may also be assessed by comparing what already exists with checklists of resources and strategies found useful elsewhere. However, it should be remembered that checklists are "closed systems", meaning that they are finite and limited to the resources and strategies that have been found useful in some locations. Not all of the criteria will apply to a given community, and there may be gaps in the checklist as far as that community is concerned. Annex 3 contains checklists for emergency preparedness.

Roles and responsibilities

Why describe roles and responsibilities?

Roles and responsibilities should be defined and described to ensure that each organization knows precisely what is expected of it and that everyone is aware of the general roles of all relevant organizations. The definition of roles and responsibilities may also assist in defusing rivalry between organizations competing for the same task or group of tasks, and will ensure that all tasks are allocated.

The following questions are relevant to the definition and description of roles and responsibilities:

- Is there an adequate description of who performs each task that is required?
- Is there an adequate description of the roles and responsibilities of each organization?
- Do members of each organization know the specific tasks to be performed by their organization?
- Do members of each organization know the general role of other organizations?
- Where is it possible to obtain the information to define and describe adequately the various roles and responsibilities?
- Which is the primary (or lead) organization for a given type of emergency, and which are the secondary (or support) organizations?

Information on roles and responsibilities

The first place to look for information on the roles and responsibilities of government organizations is legislation that describes their general functions and powers. These functions and powers are usually applicable to daily life but are also important in emergency management. For example, one of the major functions of the police is to maintain law and order, which they do every day as well as during emergencies. Government health organizations are usually involved in ensuring that steps are taken to maintain the health and well-being of the public; they will perform the same function during and after emergencies. Legislation may also provide for special organizational functions in emergency management.

NGOs often have a legislative or legal requirement to perform certain tasks. For example, industry has a responsibility to its neighbours. Any potentially harmful material in the control of an industry must be handled with sufficient care to ensure that it cannot escape and cause harm to neighbours. Potentially harmful material covers a range of possibilities, from large quantities of stored water in dams to small amounts of hazardous materials. Beyond legislation, there are likely to be interorganizational policies and agreements that affect the functions of organizations in emergency management. The resource analysis also assigns responsibilities to specific organizations for providing certain resources. Based on a vulnerability assessment and potential problem analysis, resource analysis will have determined many of the tasks required in response and recovery.

There are two suggested ways of describing roles and responsibilities: to describe them by task or to describe them by organization.

Describing roles and responsibilities by task

Describing roles and responsibilities by task assists those who want a quick overview of who is supposed to do what, and those who are responsible for controlling or coordinating emergency management activities. The description is based on a list of tasks and their allocation to the organizations. The tasks could be listed alphabetically or according to the aspect of emergency management to which they pertain, under the headings: Task, Lead organization, Support organizations.

Describing roles and responsibilities by organization
The description of roles and responsibilities by organization requires each organization to be listed and its roles described. This is useful for members of a specific organization as they can see at a glance what their organization has undertaken to do.

Assessing organizations
Organizations agree to perform certain tasks; it is therefore often necessary to assess how suitable and effective they are for an emergency response situation (5). This should be done by the planning group with all relevant organizations participating. Aspects of the assessment may include capability, availability, durability, and operational integrity.

Capability refers to whether an organization has the resources to carry out its assigned tasks. Obviously, the emergency management tasks allocated to an organization should be very similar, if not identical, to the tasks carried out by that organization under normal conditions. However, most organizations are rarely required to operate under emergency conditions, and an assessment of their ability to do so is essential.

Availability refers to how quickly an organization can apply resources in an emergency. Delays may occur because of the call-out of staff, the switching from normal activities to emergency operations, and the need to continue carrying out normal activities. Hospitals, for example, still need to treat and care for their normal patients and may rapidly become overwhelmed by an influx of new patients.

Durability refers to an organization's ability to sustain emergency operations. The size and resource base of an organization will partially determine its ability to maintain operations round the clock for many days or even weeks. Organizations will often suffer damage themselves during an emergency and may therefore be less capable than usual. Emergency situations create personal and organizational stress; if an organization is not experienced in dealing with this stress or organized to adapt to it, its durability may be affected.

Operational integrity concerns the ability of an organization to operate autonomously. In emergencies, organizations should ideally be able to accept a task, request additional resources if necessary, carry out the task, and report its successful conclusion (or any problems) to the controlling organization.

Management structure
Purpose of the management structure
The management structure defines the authority and reporting relationships between different organizations and sometimes the relationships within an organization. There should be a clear and shared understanding of these relation-

ships to minimize confusion during emergencies. Each organization involved in the plan should agree on the management structure.

Some management concepts in emergency management

A number of management concepts are commonly used in emergency management, including command, control, coordination, and lead organization.

Command directs the members and resources of an organization in performing the organization's role and tasks and operates vertically within the organization. Authority to command is established by agreement with an organization or in legislation.

Control is the overall direction of emergency activities. Authority for control is established by legislation or in a plan and carries with it the responsibility for tasking other organizations and coordinating their activities according to the needs of the situation. Control relates to situations and operates horizontally.

Coordination involves the systematic analysis of an emergency situation and available resources, and the provision of relevant information to organizations on the most effective actions to meet specific objectives.

The lead organization is the organization principally responsible for responding to a particular hazard or type of emergency.

Control of organizations during emergencies should be strategic and supportive in nature. The controller should consult with organizations as to what they should do, but should not tell them how to do it. The controller should also provide support by supplying organizations with information and resources.

In the event of an emergency occurring at the community level, local government organizations are responsible for taking appropriate action. If the scale of the emergency is such that the resources needed to control it exceed the community's capacity, the local government organization should alert and refer to the next administrative level (e.g. province, region, or country). This level should be automatically placed on the alert when several communities are affected. If several provinces are involved, or the magnitude of the emergency exceeds their coping capacity, the national plan is activated, and international aid should be sought if national resources are insufficient. Figure 21 shows the different administrative levels.

A possible management structure for the provincial level consists of a task force and six sectors. The task force comprises the director of response and recovery operations (the overall emergency controller), and the heads of each sector. The sectors are shown in Fig. 22.

The task force may be responsible for gathering, centralizing, and disseminating information, coordinating activities, and deploying staff and resources. An emergency control centre will be required during emergencies to coordinate the activities of all sectors, and a dedicated public information unit will provide

EMERGENCY PLANNING

Fig. 21. **Sequence of emergency response of different administrative levels**

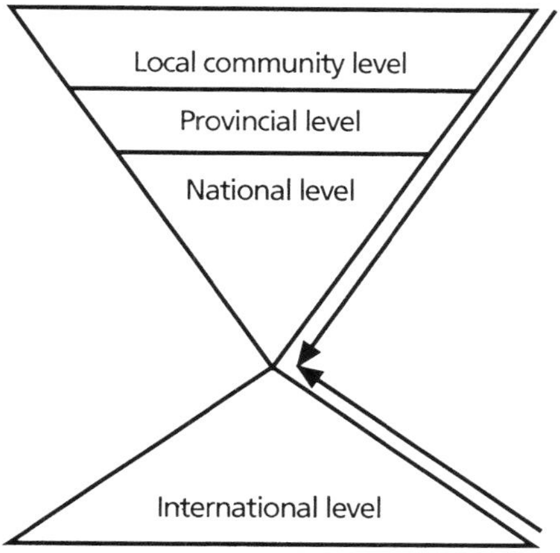

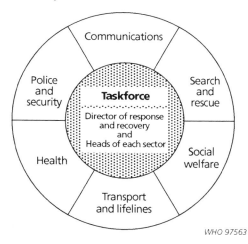

WHO 97562

Fig. 22. **A model for the multisectoral approach to emergency response and recovery**

WHO 97563

information to members of the public and to the media. Figure 23 shows such a management structure at the provincial level.

Community preparedness management structures should be designed to interface efficiently with the management structures at provincial and national levels. (See the section "Command, control, and coordination", p. 90.)

Strategies and systems

Developing strategies and systems

Strategies and systems that are commonly required for response and recovery include those for the six sectors in the model illustrated in Fig. 22, that is:

Fig. 23. **The six sectors**

Communications	**Police and security**
• *Head* Chief of provincial communications • *Role* Maintain radio and telephone contacts between organizations, including within the area of operations • *Organizations* Post and telecommunications, interior ministry, armed forces, radio amateurs, etc.	• *Head* Chief of police or national guard • *Role* Gather information and maintain public order and traffic flow, identify bodies • *Organizations* Police, national guard, customs, armed forces
Health and medical	**Search and rescue**
• *Head* Provincial director of health • *Role* Organize emergency care at emergency site, medical transport to hospitals, hospital treatment and health care for evacuees and the community • *Organizations* Health staff and resources (civilian, military, public, or private), certified first-aid workers, other services	• *Head* Chief of fire department or civil protection • *Role* Fire-fighting, rescue work, clearing rubble, protection of individuals and property • *Organizations* Fire department and other rescue services, public or private companies, railway companies, utilities (water, electricity)
Social welfare	**Transport and lifelines**
• *Head* Provincial director of social services • *Role* In cooperation with local authority (mayor, district chief, etc.) organize reception and accommodation of, and catering for, emergency victims • *Organizations* Local community services	• *Head* Provincial director of equipment and public works • *Role* Mobilize and coordinate necessary means of transport, meet special needs of other services, restore communication routes to ensure general traffic flow, restore electrical power and drinking-water supply networks • *Organizations* Public roads, road transport companies, breakdown services, repair workshops, armed forces

— communications;
— search and rescue;
— health and medical;
— social welfare;
— transport and lifelines
— police and security;

as well as:

— alerting;
— command, control, and coordination;
— information management;
— resource management;
— evacuation;
— hazardous materials.

EMERGENCY PLANNING

Aspects of each of these areas are described in this section. Reference should also be made to the checklists in Annex 3.

Communications

Communications concern the means of relaying information between organizations, individuals with particular responsibilities, and the community. Adequate communications facilities are essential to all aspects of response and recovery operations. As regards electronic communications (radio, facsimile, e-mail, etc.), the system should allow (6):

— coverage from community to provincial and national levels, both within and between organizations;
— primary reliance on existing systems and compatibility between organizations' systems;
— dedicated frequencies for command, control, and coordination;
— backup systems and backup power supplies;
— simplicity of activation and operation.

Search and rescue

The aim of search and rescue planning is to save lives and minimize further injury to people and damage to property in times of emergency. Search and rescue services, supported as necessary by specialist groups such as marine and air rescue units and mountain rescue teams, will:

— provide life-saving support to trapped people during the course of rescue operations;
— save lives by the rapid and safe extrication of trapped people;
— save lives by the rescue and recovery of people who may be at risk in difficult terrain or through abnormal weather conditions;
— recover the dead;
— provide temporary support, repair, or demolition of damaged and dangerous structures to minimize further injury to people, damage to property, or disruption to services;
— provide support, on request, to other services or specialist units.

Search and rescue planning should ensure that all people and resources engaged in search and rescue are efficiently utilized before, during, and after an emergency. It should consider three categories of rescue workers:

— survivors who are able to start immediate work at the emergency site;
— untrained personnel who usually arrive from outside the immediate area to assist the casualties;
— trained personnel who arrive in organized rescue teams and can utilize the available resources, material, and untrained personnel in carrying out life-saving tasks.

Health and medical

Health and medical planning includes:

— the broad health sector;
— public health;

- mental health;
- nutrition;
- hospital emergencies;
- the integration of rescue and medical services;
- triage and first aid.

Social welfare

Social welfare involves the care of people and the community during and after emergencies. Any emergency threatens the physical and emotional well-being of large numbers of people. Individuals may experience bereavement, physical injury, and separation from families, as well as personal losses of clothing, housing, food, household goods, employment, and income. Communities may be affected by severe damage to lifeline services (power, water, gas, electricity, and sewerage) and transport. Hence, providing for the welfare of the victims of an emergency is a fundamental task of emergency preparedness at all levels of government. Various factors such as weather, health hazards, or disruption of supplies may make it necessary to evacuate all or part of the emergency area, and planning and organization for the care of the homeless are essential to emergency preparedness.

The tasks that may be required include the provision of:

- temporary accommodation, including emergency camps;
- care of children and the elderly;
- clothing and household items;
- counselling;
- emergency feeding;
- financial assistance;
- insurance and legal advice;
- public information;
- referral service;
- registration and enquiry services.

Communities should be encouraged to manage these tasks. The natural leaders of the community should form the backbone of the emergency organization since excessive external assistance can damage a community and destroy self-reliance.

Social welfare planning should describe how people's immediate welfare needs should be met during and after an emergency and prescribe procedures to meet those needs during an evacuation and subsequent recovery. It should emphasize that social welfare is the responsibility not only of specialized government organizations, but also of all other government organizations and NGOs. Social welfare planning should set out the tasks and responsibilities of these organizations.

Past emergencies have shown that no coherent action in social welfare can be undertaken unless plans for receiving and accommodating the population are already in place. These plans should provide for human and material resources, reception areas, and intervention procedures. Ideally, plans will have been prepared well in advance and regularly updated.

As with emergency medical response, the management of emergency-stricken populations should be based on reception in two stages:

— *forward reception*, for immediate management, counting, and assessment of needs;
— *backup reception*, for temporary accommodation, family regrouping, and providing information to families.

A site outside the immediate emergency area should be selected, if possible, as the forward reception point, to avoid exposure to further accidents and to ensure that rescue operations are unhampered. The purpose is to provide immediate comfort and basic facilities for victims. There should be adequate signs and direction arrows at the reception point showing where specific resources and assistance can be found. The tasks of forward reception are thus:

— recording information on people by means of individual record cards, gathering data for reuniting families, and searching for children;
— comforting the victims, with all workers doing their part to restore psychological balance as quickly as possible and prevent further harm.

The more structured backup reception facility should be used to reunite families, with the help of the information gathered at the forward reception point. It should serve as an information coordination centre and for reorganizing the life of the community, finding and adapting accommodation, and ensuring that it is functional. This will require an inventory of the human resources and materials available, and the distribution of tasks.

Human resources

The personnel working for the backup reception should have certain technical and human skills:

- *Skills in reception and recovery.* Familiarity with the procedures and facilities for information management is essential, plus the ability to:
  — listen to people's problems, record, and classify them;
  — analyse the situation, determine the best forms of response and recovery in terms of the resources available, and rank them in order of urgency;
  — ensure that resources are used once they are distributed.
- *Technical knowledge of logistic support.* This covers areas such as energy (electricity, gas, heating, fuel), services (water, telephone), shelter, premises and their use, and catering.
- *Safety consciousness.* Personnel should be attentive to their own safety and the safety of the people in their care. They should not intervene in areas at risk.
- *Language.* Knowledge of the local language and dialects is nearly always essential for organizing response and recovery. People who speak the language should be included among the supervisory personnel.
- *Training.* Ideally, personnel should receive prior training in emergency response and recovery arrangements at the sites where they may work. It will often be necessary to rely on volunteers, who will require information and leadership from people with prior training.

- *First aid and health*. Some personnel should be capable of giving first aid. They should assist casualties who are ill or unconscious, pending the arrival of a doctor. They should carry out all necessary measures to ensure general hygiene (considering factors like presence of animals, the control of parasites, the prevention of faecal infection, etc.). In all these activities, continuous liaison with a doctor is desirable.

Material resources

Material resources may be classed as either fixed or mobile:

- *Fixed resources* — pre-arranged premises and facilities for receiving people.
- *Mobile resources* may include:
  — vehicles for transporting people and materials;
  — blankets, camp-beds;
  — sources of electric power and lighting facilities;
  — drinking-water or facilities for producing it;
  — food supplies appropriate for the population, particularly for children;
  — sheeting to cover broken windows and walls, and the means to fix it in place.

Transport and lifelines

Transport is an important factor in managing an emergency. It includes identifying and mobilizing transport resources and controlling movement. The aim of transport preparedness is to prescribe arrangements for identifying resources (road vehicles, rail, shipping, aircraft, and access routes) to ensure their best use. Planning aspects include:

— making arrangements for identifying, acquiring, or organizing public and private transport resources at every level of government;
— identifying, regulating, restoring, and maintaining access routes during an emergency;
— coordinating transport;
— ensuring compatibility with provincial and national transport planning.

An emergency is likely to disrupt lifeline services (electricity, gas, water, petroleum fuels, and communications) essential to the community's survival. Apart from its impact on the stricken area, it may affect other parts of the province or country, particularly if electricity generation, gas production capacity, or water supply systems are reduced by the emergency, or if transmission through the affected area is interrupted. Supply of other energy sources such as vehicle, aviation, and heating and cooking fuels may become irregular, or existing stocks may be destroyed.

Restoring lifeline services is an important part of re-establishing normal conditions. Those energy forms that can be supplied by road, rail, or sea transportation methods (including liquefied petroleum gas (LPG), gasoline (petrol), diesel fuel, and coal) must be dealt with in transport planning. Lifeline services planning entails strategies to restore supplies of electricity, gas, and water, etc., which are generally provided through a central supply system. In some areas, liquid gasoline (petrol) products are piped, and provincial and community emergency plans must provide for restoration of supplies in the event of disruption.

Protecting and restoring lifeline services, particularly electricity, are crucial measures in any emergency. Medical facilities, public health systems, and many other essential services depend on electricity for their continued operation, as does the commercial storage of food under refrigeration. Electricity is required for many communications systems, e.g. radio transmitters, radio-telephone systems, facsimile machines, and computer systems. Most industrial and commercial enterprises use electricity in their processes and many other buildings use it for lighting, heating, cooking, water heating, refrigeration, and air conditioning.

Gas is piped to some urban areas, and may be important for electricity generation. Failure of gas pipelines supplying power stations may reduce available electrical resources. Local power schemes, in-house and standby generators, in turn, are likely to depend on accessible stocks of LPG or diesel fuel.

The aim of lifeline services planning is to organize for the restoration, operation, and maintenance of all lifeline services under emergency conditions. It should also ensure the best use of available systems and resources in the event of an emergency, including:

— identifying electricity, gas, and water supply systems at national, provincial, and community level;
— determining what resources would be needed for restoring damaged systems and how they might be obtained during an emergency;
— ensuring that regular supplies of all services are restored as soon as possible and in order of importance;
— establishing guidelines for operational emergency plans for provincial and community organizations.

In general, the following principles should be followed in an emergency:

- Electricity supply systems should be accorded a high priority for restoration and maintenance because of their life-preserving and communications purposes.
- Piped gas supply systems should be accorded priority where they are used for fuelling power stations or where they form a major energy source for the community.
- Water supply systems should be given priority where there is possible contamination of existing supplies and where the sewerage systems are damaged and causing a risk to public health.

Police and security

An emergency creates complex problems for maintaining law and order and performing day-to-day police functions. Law and order must be maintained even during emergencies. This may prove difficult since police may be heavily committed to emergency operations. Police organizations will need to develop operational plans that ensure sufficient resources for normal policing and security.

Alerting

Alerting consists of a number of response phases, including:

- *Alert* — the period when it is believed that resources may be required, which prompts an increased level of preparedness.
- *Standby* — the period normally following an alert, when the controlling organization believes that deployment of resources is imminent and personnel are placed on standby to respond immediately.
- *Call-out* — the command to deploy resources.
- *Stand-down* — when the controlling organization declares that the emergency is controlled and that resources may be recalled.

To implement these phases, there should be:

— a protocol that stipulates which organizations to alert for which emergencies and what tasks;
— a contact list for all organizations;
— a description of the type of information that should be supplied in the various phases of alerting.

Command, control, and coordination

Command, control, and coordination concern managing people, resources, and information during response and recovery operations, and consist of the following elements:

— information management;
— resource management;
— decision-making;
— problem-solving;
— reporting to higher levels of authority.

These activities often take place in emergency coordination centres (ECCs). It is preferable to have ECCs established at national, provincial, and community levels. A model for establishing them at the provincial level is outlined below:

- The provincial ECC is established in the chief town of the province and staffed by the director of response and recovery operations (appointed by the provincial governor or prefect), representatives of the heads of the six sectors, and communications and administrative personnel.
- The operational ECC is located as close as possible to the area of operations and run by a deputy of the director of response and recovery operations and representatives of the heads of the six sectors.

The role of the provincial ECC is to:

— communicate with the operational ECC and the relevant provincial or national services;
— process information and make certain instructions are carried out;
— coordinate deployment of reinforcements or additional supplies and dispatch them to the emergency site.

The operational ECC should be located close enough to the emergency site to allow speedy and permanent liaison between the centre and personnel engaged

Table 24. **Standard operating procedures for emergency control centres**[a]

Activation	Operations	Closing-down
Open ECC	Message flow	File messages and other
Mobilize staff	Information display	documents
Activate communications systems	Information processing	Release staff
	Control resource mobilization and deployment	Close down communications
Prepare and post maps and display boards		Close down ECC
	Drafting of situation reports	Organize operational debrief
Draw up support staff roster	Decision-making	
	Briefings	
	Reporting to higher authority	

[a] Reproduced from reference 6 by permission of the publisher, Emergency Management Australia (formerly Natural Disasters Organisation).

in operations and staff on standby. It must be set up outside the danger zone and, if possible, in a building that is easy to locate — a city hall, school, or railway station, for example.

The standard operating procedures listed in Table 24 will be required for ECC operation. Individual organizations will also need to establish ECCs for their own operations.

Information management

Information management involves the gathering, handling, use, and dissemination of information related to an emergency. Tasks and systems include:

— warning systems;
— public information;
— emergency assessment.

Warning systems

Organizations responsible for emergency management should develop early-warning systems for their own use and the use of others. These early warning systems could cover the following areas:

— outbreaks of disease and epidemics;
— shortages of food;
— severe weather;
— other natural hazards;
— population movements;
— technological and industrial hazards;
— social and political unrest;
— economic crises;
— war and insurgencies.

If notification can be transmitted before an emergency strikes, the effectiveness of emergency preparedness measures can be greatly improved, especially during the early stages of the emergency. The warning system must be developed to alert the communities and emergency organizations at every level to the possible need for implementing emergency preparedness measures.

A community warning should produce appropriate responses to minimize harm. Warning messages should (6):

— provide timely information about an impending emergency;
— state the action that should be taken to reduce loss of life, injury, and property damage;
— state the consequences of failure to heed the warning;
— provide feedback to response managers on the extent of community compliance;
— cite a credible authority;
— be short, simple, and precise;
— have a personal context;
— contain active verbs;
— repeat information regularly.

Warnings should be transmitted through as many media as possible. They may be initiated in several ways: they may originate from the scene or potential scene of the emergency and be passed upwards, or they may originate from national government and be passed down to the scene of the impending emergency.

Public information

Public information in emergencies represents the deliberate, planned, and sustained effort to establish and maintain mutual understanding between those managing the response and the community. It means ensuring answers to the questions:

- What is happening?
- What should be done?
- What might happen?

Public information planning seeks to ensure that those who need the information in an emergency get it — and that those who provide the information do so in an accurate, direct, and timely way. Those who need information include:

— people who are directly affected by the emergency and have to ensure their own safety;
— people who organize the response to the emergency and prevent the situation from getting worse;
— people who disseminate public warnings and information;
— people who can contribute to an emergency response;
— people who are indirectly affected by the emergency;
— people who are interested;
— the news media.

Those who provide information include:

— people who are directly involved in the emergency and/or who organize the response to it;
— organizations with specific roles in responding to the emergency;
— the news media.

It is important to involve the news media at the planning stage of emergency preparedness. With strong, established relationships, the media can provide significant professional assistance during the response phase. When an emergency strikes, it is too late to think about planning for the role of the media.

The following are guidelines for establishing public information centres and communicating with the public.

A public information centre can be located either at a hospital or at a convenient place, not too far from the emergency area (hotel, town hall, school, etc.) or the backup reception centre. Nevertheless, it should be far enough away from where rescue activity is taking place, so that congestion and interference are reduced. The existence of such a centre and its telephone numbers should be made known through radio and television broadcasts. Families who are worried that relatives are among the victims should be invited to come to the centre. Survivors may also be asked to gather there. For several reasons, this centre can be useful when victims of an emergency die far away from their homes. It gives the bereaved a chance to meet survivors and get a first-hand report of what happened to their loved ones, how they died, and what was done to rescue them. The survivors, and possibly onlookers and rescuers, have information that often cannot be given by others. For survivors, it can be an important experience to be of help to the bereaved.

The main functions of the information centre are:

— to provide rapid, authoritative information about tragic news that can be conveyed in a humane, direct way, in a setting sheltered from public and media attention;
— to provide support and a holding environment for both survivors and helpers;
— to serve as a forum or meeting place where affected individuals and families can support each other — self-help groups may develop from this forum;
— to be a place where police can collect identification data about missing and dead people from family members;
— for use by the police to question survivors about the chain of events, as a part of their investigation;
— to help reduce the convergence of people on the emergency site, thus avoiding congestion and movement problems for rescuers.

Figure 24 shows six steps to communicating with the public.

The communication strategy should outline:

— who determines what information should be collected;
— who collects and collates information;
— who selects the information to be communicated;
— who prepares messages;
— who authorizes messages;
— who contacts the media.

An experienced media relations officer should be appointed to coordinate public information. This person should answer directly to the emergency controller or commander, and:

Fig. 24. **A process for communicating with the public**[a]

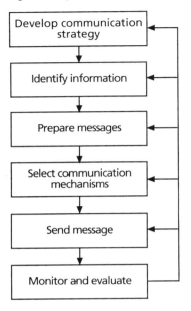

WHO 97564

[a]Reproduced from reference 7 by permission of the publisher. Enquiries about PAHO publications: paho@pmds.com

- establish contacts with key media personnel, understand how they work, brief them on his or her role, and determine how they can work together;
- communicate with the national emergency taskforce and committees;
- develop a continuous timetable for disseminating information on emergency management, including advertisements for the emergency tone (on radio and television) and symbol;
- present messages as a media package, including features, background information, and messages, with audio or video tapes when possible and appropriate.

To identify information, the information coordinator should consult with emergency management authorities to identify main issues, determine their priority, collect data, and prepare a profile of the target audience.

Prepared messages should answer the following questions:

- *Who* ... is affected, the message source, etc?
- *What* ... is the message, the problem, the solution, etc?
- *When* ... did it happen, should it happen, should there be action?
- *Where* ... what place is affected, where should people go, etc?
- *Why* ... is it important that the message be followed?
- *How* ... to respond, to deal with the situation, etc?

These messages should also:

- reassure the audience;
- capture the audience's attention through the use of an emergency tone, symbols, etc.
- use "catchy" wording and be conversational in tone and choice of words, be clear in whatever language is used, and avoid technical jargon;
- say where further information and help can be obtained;
- be concise (lasting 15–60 seconds);
- give accurate (technically sound) information;
- be current;
- use prominent personalities to endorse and give credibility to the messages;
- state specifically and precisely what behaviour is required, what is expected, what must be done.

When selecting communication mechanisms and sending messages, it is advisable to use a variety of media, such as television, radio, newspapers, newsletters, posters, amateur radio, public address systems, government personnel, and volunteers. Communications could include:

- news releases;
- public service announcements;
- talk shows, including call-in programmes;
- advertisements;
- flyers, circulars;
- local community personnel — emergency management committee members, service clubs, voluntary organizations, and police and fire department officers.

Key messages and important releases should be broadcast at prime time, usually 6:00–8:00 and 17:00–19:00 in most countries. Electronic and print media have news deadlines: the information coordinator should discuss these with media personnel and determine the best times of day for media releases. Representatives of other media should be informed of the time and place of releases and briefings. If the media are supplied with accurate, complete information, on time, they will be of great assistance in emergency response and recovery.

Before messages are sent to the media, they should be tested on a sample audience to ensure that they have exactly the desired effect.

Monitoring and evaluation should focus on the effectiveness, efficiency, and appropriateness of the public communication strategy and provide information for improving it. This can be done through:

- simulation exercises;
- monitoring media messages before and during emergencies;
- surveys;
- questionnaires;
- formal reviews after emergencies.

Emergency assessment

The critical component of any emergency response is the early conduct of an emergency assessment to identify urgent needs and to determine response and recovery priorities. An emergency assessment provides response and recovery managers with information about the effects of the emergency on the population. This information is collected by rapidly conducted field investigations. The early completion of this task and subsequent mobilization of resources to address the urgent needs of the affected population can significantly reduce the adverse consequences of an emergency. Inadequate assessment of human needs at the emergency site leads to inappropriate and delayed response and recovery services.

Assessment is the process of determining (8):

— the impact that an emergency has had on a community;
— the needs and priorities for immediate emergency action to save and maintain life;
— the resources available;
— possible strategies for long-term recovery and development.

Figure 25 shows how emergency assessment objectives evolve over time and Figure 26 shows an assessment process.

It is essential to distinguish between *data* and *information* — data are facts and figures, information is the interpreted data that can be used to support ideas and opinions. Much of the data that may be collected on emergencies may be irrelevant, so it is necessary to collect data that are immediately useful. This will require planning before the event and monitoring during the event. An assessment plan should outline the assessment's objectives, type of information required, means of data collection, analysis, and interpretation, and frequency of reporting.

Fig. 25. **Evolving objectives of assessment**[a]

Warning
- Determine action being taken by community to protect lives and facilities from expected emergency
- Activate the implementation of assessment

Emergency
- Confirm the reported emergency and estimate overall magnitude of the harm
- Identify, characterize, and quantify "populations at risk"
- Help to identify and prioritize the actions and resources needed to reduce immediate risks
- Identify local response capacity, including organizational, medical, and logistic resources
- Help anticipate future serious problems
- Help manage and control the immediate response

Short-term recovery
- Identify the affected community
- Identify the policies of the government with regard to recovery
- Estimate the additional support required from provincial, national, and international sources for recovery
- Monitor the outcome and effectiveness of recovery strategies

Long-term recovery
- Determine the damage to economically significant resources and the implications for development policy
- Assess the impact of the emergency on current development programmes
- Identify new development opportunities created by the emergency

WHO 97565

[a] Adapted from reference *8* by permission of the publisher.

Fig. 26. **The assessment process**[a]

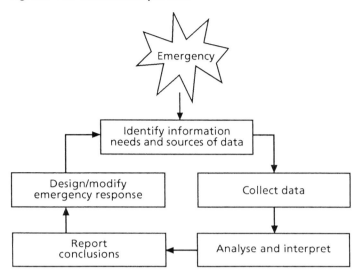

[a] Reproduced from reference 8 by permission of the publisher.

The information needs will be the gap between the data already to hand and the data required to form a reliable picture of the situation. Hence, the data already acquired will need to be verified, and geographical or functional areas for which there is no information checked. The community vulnerability assessment is a guide to where harm may have occurred and its seriousness, and can be used to check the completeness of existing data.

Sources of data could be the normal local channels (if they have not been disrupted), specific survey teams, or visual inspection by vehicle or aircraft.

Analysis and interpretation involve assessing the value, reliability, and accuracy of data, validating them against known facts, and incorporating them into a meaningful picture.

Reporting should be to those responsible for emergency response and recovery to allow modification of operations.

Information to collect during an emergency assessment of an emergency site might include (9):

— geographical extent of the impact of the emergency;
— population affected or at risk;
— presence of continuing hazards;
— injuries and deaths;
— availability of shelter;
— access to potable water;

— nutritional status of affected population;
— current level of sanitation;
— status of health-care infrastructure;
— extent and capacity of communications network;
— status of transportation system;
— incidence of communicable disease.

The assessment team should focus on problems that have potential solutions and affect the largest number of people. An imprecise knowledge of the affected population's characteristics and of ongoing hazards (e.g. toxic substances or fires) makes it more difficult to conduct an emergency assessment rapidly. In addition, logistic problems and severe time constraints make it impractical to evaluate the urgent needs of every person who has been affected by the emergency. For expediency, emergency assessment is usually conducted by sampling the needs of carefully chosen subpopulations believed to represent the needs of the entire affected population. Individuals or groups of people are surveyed rapidly in a systematic fashion to ascertain the extent of their emergency needs. Usually, this is done by directly interviewing or evaluating emergency victims, or by data abstraction at response and recovery facilities that serve populations affected by an emergency. In many emergencies there may appear to be a disproportionately high number of households headed by women.

At the emergency site, assessment personnel should attempt to survey a cross-section of the affected population (e.g. a mix of rural and urban, young and old, near and remote). This is because all areas within a region may not be affected uniformly by an emergency. Some areas may contain populations so severely affected that they are rendered completely inaccessible and silent because local roads and communication systems have been destroyed. On the other hand, areas with relatively minor damage are consistently able to convey graphic images of highly localized destruction to the response and recovery organizations, potentially diverting attention and resources from more devastated regions. In addition, a population with a homogeneous exposure to an emergency may have subpopulations that are more severely affected. Experience with refugee and displaced populations has shown disproportionately high levels of morbidity and relatively high crude mortality rates among the very young. This is the result of the effects of poor nutrition and infectious disease often found in this subpopulation under such circumstances. An emergency assessment that surveyed only the male heads of household in such circumstances might fail to identify, or direct resources to, this vulnerable subpopulation.

The specific information collected and the sampling strategy employed during an emergency depend on the nature of the emergency. During a sudden-impact emergency, the initial assessment should be completed within 24–48 hours. Slow-onset emergencies, such as droughts, famines, or other situations that create displaced or refugee populations, may not be recognized as emergencies for several months. In such circumstances, public health officials should make a baseline assessment and institute long-term surveillance. This surveillance, designed to monitor the effectiveness of response and recovery activities as well as changes in the affected population's status, may be the most important task for the assessment team. The relative importance of parts of the assessment to the overall assessment depends on the type of emergency and on other environmental factors, such as climate and geography. For example, the emergency assessment priorities related to the type of emergency are as follows:

Sudden-impact emergencies	*Gradual-onset emergencies*
Ongoing hazards	Mortality rates
Injuries and deaths	Nutritional status
Shelter requirements	Immunization status
Potable water	Environmental health

Emergency assessment rarely needs to be complicated to be of great value in determining emergency response priorities. Many standardized questionnaires and survey techniques exist to guide the field activities of assessment personnel. A coordinated approach to the assessment task will facilitate communications between managers of response and recovery operations and assessment personnel. Emergency assessment protocols can be easily incorporated into emergency preparedness and response activities at the local level and are highly effective when integrated in this manner. This is extremely important since the local community remains the principal unit in preparedness, mitigation, and response, despite the recent development of a massive international response and recovery network.

Flights over the emergency site and meetings with officials rarely provide an accurate and timely summation of the needs of the affected population. Consistently, a relatively small amount of key information, rapidly collected on-site from representative populations, concerning sentinel events or health conditions (e.g. death, illness, and injuries) will provide adequate public health intelligence upon which to base emergency response and recovery operations. Despite advances in technology and transportation, this task remains a labour-intensive field exercise, drawing upon a wide range of skills.

Information on rapid health assessment can be found in the WHO publication *Rapid health assessment protocols for emergencies* (*9*). The objectives of rapid health assessment are to:

— confirm the emergency;
— describe the type, impact, and possible evolution of the emergency;
— measure its present and potential health impact;
— assess the adequacy of existing response capacity and immediate additional needs;
— recommend priority action for immediate response.

WHO's *Rapid health assessment protocols for emergencies* describes the basic techniques and information including:

— assembling the assessment team;
— carrying out the assessment;
— important considerations;
— common sources of error;
— presentation of results and reporting;
— techniques for surveys during rapid assessment;
— preparedness for emergencies.

Resource management

A major emergency or disaster creates special resource management problems. Arrangements essential to regular supply, such as transportation routes, communications networks, and financial systems through normal credit facilities, may be disrupted or threatened. Existing stocks of essential supplies may have been damaged or destroyed. The supply requirements may thus grow at precisely the time when the means of supply have diminished. The emergency will also create demands for additional resources, including machinery and materials to rebuild and repair facilities, fuel for machinery, and food. These resources will be required not only by those stricken by the emergency but also by those involved in the recovery work.

Resource management planning for emergencies is likely to focus on the needs of rescue, medical, welfare, and recovery services forming part of the emergency response effort but should not neglect the continuing needs of the community. Without an efficient supply system, the response to the emergency and the recovery of the local community and economy will be severely hampered. Emergency plans must therefore establish an emergency resource management organization in advance of an emergency, and supply and procurement procedures that will operate once an emergency appears imminent or occurs. Possible disruptions to the local economy and the effects on the community's welfare must be considered in this planning and, if necessary, measures prepared to overcome them.

Resource management planning must cover:

— the principles of supply in an emergency, including the selection, procurement, distribution, use, and pre-positioning of essential stockpiles;
— the roles and responsibilities of organizations at all levels in providing supply systems in the event of emergency;
— the procedures that should be established for the proper accounting of resources obtained under this plan.

If specialist equipment is to be used, it is essential to ensure that the equipment is accompanied by a trained operator.

No matter what the emergency or the condition of the community, resources should always be sought at the community level first. This is not purely for reasons of cost and efficiency: the swamping of a community with excessive outside resources can:

— bankrupt local businesses;
— destroy local pride and self-sufficiency;
— lead to an unnatural degree of dependence on regional, national, and international resources;
— increase vulnerability.

The management of supplies from external sources after an emergency can be accomplished using a system known as the "Supply Management Project in the Aftermath of Disasters", otherwise known as SUMA. SUMA is a systematic approach to identifying supplies received, using trained personnel and computer software to manage response and recovery supplies and the sorting process during an emergency. This system has been developed for supplies received from outside an emergency-affected country and is currently being used at the subnational level.

There are also a number of published lists of medical and other resources that can assist in satisfying some of the material needs of emergency-affected communities.

A basic kit of materials for health emergencies is described in *The new emergency health kit 1998* (*10*). The lists of materials are based on epidemiological research on displaced populations, and the kits have been field-tested in a variety of emergency conditions. The lists consist of drugs and medical supplies that can be used to satisfy the basic medical needs of 10 000 people for approximately 3 months.

When assembled the kits weigh 860 kg and occupy $4 \, m^3$, which means that they can be transported en masse in a small truck. To allow the appropriate distribution of drugs and medical supplies, and to allow the kit to be transported by means other than truck, the kit can be packaged as separate units.

- There are 10 basic units, each weighing 45 kg, which are intended for use by basic health workers for populations of 1000. They contain drugs, renewable supplies, and basic equipment.
- There is one supplementary unit for physicians and senior health workers, for a population of 10 000, containing drugs, essential infusions, renewable supplies, and equipment. This kit contains no material that is in the basic unit, and must be used *with* the basic units.

Resupply of drugs and medical supplies following the receipt of a health kit should be based on actual need, rather than requests for complete kits.

Stockpiles of emergency response and recovery supplies or requests for such supplies can be based on the publication *Emergency relief items: compendium of generic specifications* (*11*). This publication, in two volumes, specifies the most suitable resources for emergency response and recovery, and could provide guidance and assistance to:

— donor and recipient governments and institutions concerned with planning, budgeting, and the execution of assistance in emergency situations;
— procurement officials of the United Nations system, and NGOs and development agencies involved in acquiring emergency response and recovery items.

The first volume contains equipment specifications and provides guidance on needs and recommended responses for:

— telecommunications equipment;
— shelter, housing, storage, and cooking appliances;
— water supply systems;

— food items;
— sanitation and hygiene items;
— materials handling equipment;
— power supply systems.

A chapter on logistics appears at the end of the first volume, providing guidance on packaging, quality inspection, selection of mode of transport and shipping arrangements, and insurance. The second volume contains specifications for medical supplies and equipment, including essential drugs.

Descriptions of emergency kits for a variety of purposes can be found in *Guide of kits and emergency items* (*12*). These kits are grouped under the following headings:

— medical kits;
— medical modules;
— surgical instruments sets;
— logistic kits;
— miscellaneous emergency items.

Drugs are one of the most important and sensitive resources in emergency response and recovery. Both donors and recipient nations should develop policies and procedures for drug management, based on the following core donation principles (*13*):

— maximum benefit to the recipient;
— respect for the wishes and authority of the recipient;
— no double standards in quality;
— effective communication between donor and recipient.

There are 12 guidelines for drug donations:

1. All drug donations should be based on an expressed need and be relevant to the disease pattern in the recipient country. Drugs should not be sent without prior consent of the recipient.
2. All donated drugs or their generic equivalents should be approved for use in the recipient country and appear on the national list of essential drugs or, if a national list is not available, on the WHO Model List of Essential Drugs, unless specifically requested otherwise by the recipient.
3. The presentation, strength, and formulation of donated drugs should, as much as possible, be similar to those commonly used in the recipient country.
4. All donated drugs should be obtained from a reliable source and comply with quality standards in both donor and recipient country. The WHO Certification Scheme on the Quality of Pharmaceutical Products Moving in International Commerce (*14*) should be used.
5. No drugs should be donated that have been issued to patients and then returned to a pharmacy or elsewhere, or that were given to health professionals as free samples.
6. After arrival in the recipient country, all donated drugs should have a remaining shelf-life of at least one year.
7. All drugs should be labelled in a language that is easily understood by health professionals in the recipient country. The label on each individual container

should at least contain the international nonproprietary name (INN, or generic name), batch number, dosage form, strength, name of manufacturer, quantity in the container, storage conditions and expiry date.
8. As much as possible, donated drugs should be presented in larger-quantity units and hospital packs.
9. All drug donations should be packed in accordance with international shipping regulations, and be accompanied by a detailed packing list that specifies the contents of each numbered carton by INN, dosage form, quantity, batch number, expiry date, volume, weight, and any special storage conditions. The weight per carton should not exceed 50 kg. Drugs should not be mixed with other supplies in the same carton.
10. Recipients should be informed of all drug donations that are being considered, have been prepared, or are actually underway.
11. In the recipient country the declared value of a drug donation should be based upon the wholesale price of its generic equivalent in that country, or, if such information is not available, on the wholesale world-market price for its generic equivalent.
12. Costs of international and local transport, warehousing, port clearance, and appropriate storage and handling should be paid by the donor agency, unless specifically agreed otherwise with the recipient in advance.

To manage drug donations, a country should (*13*):

- Define national guidelines for drug donations and provide them to prospective donors.
- Define administrative procedures for receiving drug donations that answer the following questions:
  — Who is responsible for defining the needs, and who will prioritize them?
  — Who coordinates all drug donations?
  — Which documents are needed when a donation is planned? Who should receive them?
  — Which procedure is used when donations do not follow the guidelines?
  — What are the criteria for accepting or rejecting a donation? Who makes the final decision?
  — Who coordinates reception, storage, and distribution of the donated drugs?
  — How are donations valued and entered into the budget expenditure records?
  — How will inappropriate donations be disposed of?
- Specify the needs for donated drugs, indicating the required quantities, prioritizing the items, and stating donations already in the pipeline or expected.
- Manage donated drugs carefully by inspection upon arrival, confirmation to donor of arrival, storage and distribution by trained professionals, and accounting of receipts and distribution to ensure the drugs are used for their original purpose.

Evacuation

Evacuation is itself a hazard, in that it may place members of a community in some danger, and will remove them from their familiar surroundings under stressful circumstances (*5*). Evacuation is not a one-way trip — arrangements are required for returning evacuated people to their homes. The likely stages of evacuation are warning, withdrawal, shelter and feeding, reunion, and return. The following will need to be identified:

— assembly area sites;
— evacuation centre or reception sites;
— evacuation routes and alternatives;
— organizations responsible for assisting evacuation;
— teams for the registration of evacuees;
— transport arrangements;
— means of operating evacuation centres.

Hazardous materials

Hazardous materials include at least those listed in Table A2.9 (Dangerous goods classes) in Annex 2, that is:

— explosives;
— gases — compressed, liquefied, or dissolved under pressure;
— flammable liquids;
— flammable solids;
— oxidizing agents and organic peroxides;
— poisonous (toxic) and infectious substances;
— radioactive substances;
— corrosives.

These materials may give rise to emergencies or be involved in emergencies caused by other means. When contained, stored, used, or disposed of in appropriate ways, these materials are not harmful, but when released, burnt, damaged, etc. they may be dangerous to people, property, and the environment.

The following preparedness actions are required for a community, building, or organization to reduce the possible harm caused by hazardous materials:

- Reduce the quantity of hazardous materials stored to the minimum — the fewer materials stored, the less harm may be caused.
- Ensure that the production, storage, transport, use, and disposal of hazardous materials are carried out according to the relevant standards and are regularly audited.
- Allow only trained people to handle hazardous materials.
- Maintain an inventory of hazardous materials types, quantities, and locations.
- Collect, and have available, safety data sheets on all materials; these describe the nature of the materials, the hazards associated with them, and emergency response and first-aid directions.
- Develop generic hazardous materials emergency plans for communities and regions.

Content of community emergency plans

The content of a community emergency plan depends on:

— the hazards the community faces;
— the types of community vulnerability;

- the culture of the community;
- the means of organizing emergency management chosen by the community;
- the organization of emergency management at the provincial and national levels.

Table 25 shows some possible elements of a community emergency plan.

Table 25. **Possible content of a community emergency response and recovery plan**

Chapter	Section	Content
1. Introduction	• Aim, objectives, scope, authority • Related documents • Definitions and abbreviations • Vulnerability assessment	 • (refer to appendix) • (refer to appendix) • (refer to appendix)
2. Management structure	• Emergency powers • Control • Command • Communication • Emergency coordination centres • Post-emergency review	• Powers to release or commandeer resources • Relationship between organizations and organizational levels • Management of ECCs • Management of debriefs and review
3. Organization roles	• Description by role • Description by organization • Emergency control centres (ECCs)	• Description of roles and responsibilities • Management of ECCs
4. Information management	• Alerting • Damage assessment • Information processing • Public information • Reporting • Translation and interpretation	• Means of gathering information • Means of handling information • Types of information released • Reporting to higher authorities • Language interpretation
5. Resource management	• Resource coordination • Administration • Financial procedures • External assistance (provincial, national, and international)	• Resource analysis • Resource deployment and monitoring • Accounting for expenditure
6. Specific plans	• Search and rescue • Evacuation • Health and medical • Social welfare • Hazardous materials • Transport and lifelines • Police and security	• Specific plans of action for specific aspects of response and recovery
Appendices	• Issue history and amendment list • Distribution list • Definitions and abbreviations • Summary of vulnerability assessment • Maps • Planning groups • Emergency contacts	• Means of distributing and maintaining the emergency plan • Short list of essential terms and abbreviations, and their meanings • Description of likely effects of emergencies • Hazard, community, and vulnerability maps • Names and contact details of relevant people and organizations

Summary

- Emergency planning should be based on an assessment of vulnerability.
- An emergency plan is an agreed set of arrangements for responding to and recovering from emergencies; it describes responsibilities, management structures, strategies, and resources.
- The emergency planning process can be applied to any community, organization, or activity.
- The process of planning is as important as a written emergency plan.
- Emergency planning should be performed by an appropriate planning group.
- Potential problem analysis can determine problems, causes, preventive strategies, response and recovery strategies, and trigger events.
- The resources required to support preparedness and response and recovery strategies should be analysed.
- The roles and responsibilities of people and organizations must be defined and described.
- A management structure for emergency response and recovery should be developed based on normal management structures.
- A series of strategies and systems must be developed for response and recovery, including:
  — communications;
  — search and rescue;
  — health and medical;
  — social welfare;
  — transport and lifelines;
  — police and security;
  — alerting;
  — command, control, and coordination;
  — information management;
  — resource management;
  — evacuation;
  — hazardous materials.

References

1. Dynes R, Quarantelli E, Kreps G. *A perspective on disaster planning.* Columbus, OH, Disaster Research Center, Ohio State University, 1972.

2. Brown CA, Graham WJ. Assessing the threat to life from dam failure. *Water resources bulletin*, 1988, 24(6):1303–1309.

3. McLaughlin DA. Framework for integrated emergency management. *Public administration review*, 1985, 45:169–176.

4. *Project management.* Princeton, NJ, Kepner-Tregoe, 1987.

5. Carter WN. *Disaster management: a disaster manager's handbook.* Manila, Asian Development Bank, 1991.

6. *Australian emergency manual: community emergency planning guide*, 2nd ed. Canberra, Natural Disasters Organisation, 1992.

7. *Communication with the public in times of disaster — guidelines for disaster managers on preparing and disseminating effective health messages.* Washington, DC, Pan American Health Organization, 1994.

8. Stephenson RS. *Disaster assessment — disaster management training programme.* United Nations Development Programme/Office of the United Nations Disaster Relief Coordinator, 1991.

9. *Rapid health assessment protocols for emergencies.* Geneva, World Health Organization, 1999.

10. *The new emergency health kit 1998.* Geneva, World Health Organization, 1998 (unpublished WHO document WHO/DAP/98.10, available on request from Action Programme on Essential Drugs, World Health Organization, 1211 Geneva 27, Switzerland).

11. *Emergency relief items: compendium of generic specifications.* New York, United Nations Development Programme, 1995.

12. *Guide of kits and emergency items.* Amsterdam, Médecins Sans Frontières, 1995.

13. *Guidelines for drug donations.* Geneva, World Health Organization, 1996 (unpublished WHO document WHO/DAP/96.2, available on request from Action Programme on Essential Drugs, World Health Organization, 1211 Geneva 27, Switzerland).

14. *WHO Expert Committee on Specifications for Pharmaceutical Preparations. Thirty-fourth report.* Geneva, World Health Organization, 1996 (WHO Technical Report Series, No. 863).

Chapter 5
Training and education

Introduction

The objectives of training and education in emergency management are to:

— make the community aware of the hazards that face it;
— empower the community to participate in developing emergency management strategies;
— make the community aware of appropriate actions for different types of emergencies, and the organizations to which it can turn for assistance;
— enable emergency management personnel to carry out the tasks allotted to them.

A number of possible training and education strategies are suitable for different audiences and purposes. Strategy selection should be based on need, audience, purpose, and available time, money, and other resources. Training and education strategies may include (*1*):

— workshops, seminars, formal education programmes, or conferences;
— self-directed learning;
— individual tuition;
— exercises;
— pamphlets, videos, media advertisements, newsletters or journals;
— informal or formal presentations;
— public displays or public meetings.

This chapter describes a systematic approach to training useful for emergency management personnel and the development of public education strategies.

A systematic approach to training

The systems approach to training is a process for developing appropriate, effective, and efficient training programmes. Table 26 summarizes the steps in the process.

Analysing training needs

The objectives of the training needs analysis in emergency management are to:

— describe allocated tasks;
— determine those tasks that an organization's personnel are capable of undertaking;
— determine which personnel require further training.

For any task there are desirable levels of skills and knowledge that will ensure that it will be performed correctly. Techniques for determining desirable levels of knowledge and skill may include (*1*):

- identifying competence required;
- vulnerability assessment;
- emergency planning;
- exercises;
- analysis of emergency operations.

Techniques for determining existing levels of knowledge and skill may include (*1*):

- skills audit;
- exercises;
- analysis of emergency operations.

A comparison between desirable and existing levels of knowledge and skill will indicate the training needs.

Table 26. **The systems approach to training**[a]

Steps	Activities	Outputs
1. Analyse training need	• The job is analysed and task performances, together with task conditions and standards, are listed • Training needs, and their priorities, are listed	• A list of task performances, conditions, and standards • A schedule of training and priorities
2. Design training	• Training is designed to suit the results of job analysis • Training objectives and assessments are written and placed in logical sequence	• Sequenced set of training objectives and tests
3. Develop instruction	• Instructional methods and media are chosen • Course programme and content are compiled • The instruction is trialled and amended until it is successful	• A programme of instruction has been successfully trialled
4. Conduct instruction	• The course is conducted • Tests are administered • Initial problems are remedied	• Trainees who have achieved course objectives • A course modified as necessary
5. Validate training	• Problem areas from 4 and 5 are identified by analysing: — efficiency — whether best use was made of resources to achieve objectives — effectiveness — whether skills and knowledge were increased — appropriateness — the relevance of the training received to the job • Training is modified or updated as necessary	• Validated and successful training

[a] Reproduced from reference *2* by permission of the publisher, Emergency Management Australia (formerly Natural Disasters Organisation).

Designing training

Training should be based on needs. To design appropriate training it is necessary to develop training objectives that are mandatory, measurable, realistic, and achievable. Training objectives describe the performance required in tasks, and therefore describe what a course participant should be able to do. For example, training objectives in an emergency management course may be based on participants learning to:

— explain how to form an appropriate emergency planning group;
— lead a group in identifying hazards;
— apply a number of methods for describing hazards, the community, and community vulnerability.

Assessment can take a number of forms, such as:

— observation in the workplace by a supervisor;
— demonstration in a structured and practical manner;
— project-based assessment where a relevant project is undertaken on an unsupervised basis;
— simulation of the task, including role-play;
— structured tests (either written multiple-choice, short answer, extended answer, or oral);
— continual assessment of work-based performance.

Developing and conducting instruction

A training or education plan should be developed containing:

— a summary of training and education objectives;
— a programme;
— allocation of responsibility;
— resource requirements;
— delivery modes;
— assessment, validation, and evaluation processes.

Validating training

To validate training, instruments should be developed and implemented for:

— assessment;
— validation;
— evaluation.

Assessment is the measurement of an individual's current knowledge, skills, and competence, and is a baseline for measuring the effectiveness of training. Techniques may include practical assessment, on-the-job assessment, and examination. Assessment can be performed before and after training.

Validation is the comparison between the outcomes achieved by training and education and the desired outcomes, which determines the appropriateness of the training.

Evaluation is the process of determining the efficiency and effectiveness of a training and education plan. Part of the process is the comparison of outputs and objectives.

Public education

> "The aim of public education is to ensure an alert and informed community. There is a requirement to have the community informed about the characteristics and possible effects of identified hazards. Public education material needs to contain action statements which will direct the public to make desired preparations and take appropriate actions. . . . particular attention is given to identified special needs groups. A broad range of methods for dissemination should be considered, including:
>
> — newspapers;
> — radio;
> — television;
> — brochures;
> — public meetings;
> — school visits.
>
> It is also useful to advertise the existence of hazard analysis and emergency plans, and to place these on public view." (3)

Annex 4 contains information that can be provided to communities on personal protection in different types of emergencies.

Summary

The objectives of training and education in emergency management are to:

— make the community aware of the hazards that face it;
— empower the community to participate in developing emergency management strategies;
— make the community aware of appropriate actions for different types of emergencies and the organizations to which it can turn for assistance;
— enable emergency management personnel to carry out the tasks allotted to them.

A systematic approach to training is a process for developing appropriate, effective, and efficient training programmes, involving:

— analysing training needs;
— designing training;
— developing instruction;
— conducting instruction;
— validating training.

Public education programmes should be conducted to ensure an alert and informed community.

References

1. *National emergency management competency standards.* Canberra, Emergency Management Australia, 1995.

2. *Australian emergency manual: training management.* Canberra, Natural Disasters Organisation, 1992.

3. *Australian emergency manual: community emergency planning guide*, 2nd ed. Canberra, Natural Disasters Organisation, 1992.

Chapter 6
Monitoring and evaluation

Introduction

Monitoring and evaluation determine how well an emergency preparedness programme is being developed and implemented and what needs to be done to improve it. The method can be applied to:

— developing and implementing policy;
— vulnerability assessment;
— emergency planning;
— organizational preparedness;
— training and education.

Three ways of monitoring and evaluating preparedness are described here:

— project management;
— checklists;
— exercises.

Project management

The means of monitoring and evaluating during the implementation phase of a project include: measuring the progress toward project objectives; performing an analysis to find the cause of deviations in the project; and determining corrective actions. (See Annex 1 for more details.)

Projects involve analysing the present and past, predicting the future, making changes, and developing new ideas and products for future use. Very often the analyses, predictions, changes, and new ideas and products are not entirely correct, and over time the environment in which the project is being implemented will change. In each part of the emergency preparedness process described in this manual it is possible to make mistakes, and there is always room for improvement.

Policies describe long-term goals and assign responsibilities, and may establish work practices and decision criteria. It is possible, however, that a policy goal may be set too high to be achieved or be incorrect in other ways. Policy review cannot be continuous, or the basis for all emergency management programmes would be continually altering and individual projects would not be completed. Policy-makers should remain receptive to criticism and suggestions, and should periodically review policies in the light of experience, changes in the policy and emergency management environment, and new challenges that arise, remembering that policy development is a participatory process. If a policy is embodied in legislation, a common reaction to suggestions for change is "But we can't, it's the law!" Laws are made to be useful and can be changed when they no longer serve their purpose.

Vulnerability assessment can determine community vulnerabilities, describe hazards and the harm they may cause, and provide information for all aspects of emergency management. The accuracy of a vulnerability assessment is determined by the quality of:

— community participation;
— the information used;
— the resources applied;
— the assumptions about the community, the environment, and the hazards;
— the conceptual models.

Vulnerability assessment will never present a perfectly correct picture of vulnerability, hazards, and potential emergencies. When an emergency has occurred, it is often discovered that the models used to describe the behaviour of a hazard are incorrect. For example, actual floods rarely follow precisely the flood heights and time scales predicted. The models therefore need to be fine-tuned. Assumptions about community vulnerability sometimes prove unfounded, and predictions of community behaviour during emergencies are not always correct. Thus, the analysis of emergencies — even minor ones that cause little harm — can yield information that will make a vulnerability assessment more accurate.

There is also inevitable change in the community, environment, and vulnerability. Effective vulnerability reduction and emergency preparedness programmes will create changes for the better, and economic, environmental, and social influences may create changes for the worse. Thus, vulnerability assessment needs to be reviewed periodically.

Emergency planning is intended to protect the community and its environment, and to reduce uncertainty and confusion during emergencies. Sometimes emergency plans do not work. One of the most common reasons for this is that plans were developed in isolation and not communicated to the right people. Other reasons may include:

— poor communication (both technical and personal) during the emergency;
— lack of coordination of response work, leading to duplication, inefficiency, and ineffectiveness;
— lack of resources for the problems at hand.

After each emergency, an analysis of the events and actions that occurred is required. Each organization involved should hold debriefings, and then there should be a single debriefing for representatives of all organizations. A debriefing entails presenting facts of the emergency, describing the role that each person or organization played, and evaluating the actions taken. While debriefings are instructive for those who participate, they should also be documented and used to improve emergency planning.

Checklists

Checklists can be used to evaluate an existing emergency preparedness programme or to assist in developing a new programme. Checklists constitute a "closed set" in that they are not tools for developing new ideas or strategies. They can, however, form a compendium of current knowledge based on prior experience, and they are simple and easy to use.

Annex 3 contains a number of checklists for emergency preparedness, as well as for response and recovery. These checklists are not exhaustive, and can be added to as experience is gained or to suit the context of a community's preparedness.[1]

Exercises

A common way of monitoring and evaluating parts of an emergency preparedness programme is through conducting exercises, which can be used to test aspects of:

— emergency plans;
— emergency procedures;
— training;
— communications, etc.

There are many different types of exercise, each suited to different purposes. The purpose of an exercise, and the aspect of emergency preparedness to be tested, must be carefully decided and fairly specific. An exercise should not be conducted with the purpose of testing an entire emergency plan or all aspects of training. Some specific purposes for exercises related to communications include:

— to test the communications procedures contained within an organization's emergency procedures;
— to validate the interorganization communications covered in a plan;
— to test the call-out procedures within an organization;
— to validate the lines of command and control defined by a plan;
— to test the ability of organizations to establish and maintain emergency operations centres;
— to test the response times of organizations involved in a plan.

Some typical types of exercise include the following:

- *Operational exercise*, in which personnel and resources are deployed in a simulation of an emergency.
- *Tabletop exercise*, in which personnel are presented with an unfolding scenario, asked what actions would be required, and how the actions would be implemented.
- *Syndicate exercise*, in which personnel are divided into syndicates to discuss and consider a given scenario, and the syndicate planning and response decisions are then discussed in an open forum.

There are also a number of different ways of organizing, conducting, and reviewing exercises. One way is to go through the following steps.

[1] Further information on assessing health sector emergency preparedness can be found in *Guidelines for assessing disaster preparedness in the health sector*, Washington, DC, Pan American Health Organization, 1995.

- Determine need. Exercises can be expensive and time-consuming, and sometimes dangerous. There must be a clear need for the exercise, and it must be targeted appropriately. An exercise writing team should be formed to define and design the exercise.
- Define exercise. This involves determining:
  — the aim, objectives, and scope of the exercise;
  — type of exercise;
  — the authority for its conduct;
  — the performance standards that will be used to judge the degree of success of the exercise;
  — organizations to be involved;
  — resources and budget.
- Design exercise. Exercise design involves determining:
  — appropriate exercise scenario(s);
  — any special aids that may be required;
  — timelines;
  — exercise appointments;
  — exercise control;
  — safety requirements.
- Conduct exercise.
- Conduct exercise debriefing. The debriefing should be a meeting of those involved in the exercise to consider the degree of success in meeting the performance standards and in achieving the objectives;
- Validate exercise. This involves determining how plans, procedures, and training can be improved on the basis of the exercise results.

Selection of exercise writing team

Some of the criteria for selecting members of an exercise writing team include:

- At least one member should have some expertise in exercise writing.
- If a number of organizations are participating, each of the major organizations should be represented.
- Members should have experience in the areas to be tested or validated.
- The chairperson of the writing team should be from the lead organization.

Exercise appointments

To ensure effective exercise control, exercise control personnel should include:

  — an exercise director;
  — an exercise administrator;
  — exercise umpires or directing staff;
  — visitor or media liaison officer.

For operational exercises, the following appointments may also be necessary:

  — damage control officers;
  — safety officers;
  — scenario coordinators.

Summary

- Monitoring and evaluation involves determining how well an emergency preparedness programme is being developed and implemented, and what needs to be done to improve it.
- Three ways of monitoring and evaluating preparedness are:
  — project management;
  — checklists;
  — exercises.

Annex 1
Project management

There are three major parts to project management: definition, planning, and implementation (*1*).

Project definition

The project definition determines the project's aim and objectives as well as its scope, authority, and context. In addition to providing a brief outline to others of the project's intentions, the project definition gives a description of the project for those from whom funding may be sought. A project manager should be appointed to manage the project.

The aim is a statement explaining the project's purpose. This should be a single-sentence statement describing the desired end result or outcome. Objectives are what must be achieved in order to satisfy the aim — they are the tangible outputs of the project. The objectives of the project should be:

- achievable and realistic (within the constraints of the project);
- mandatory (if a specific objective is not achieved, then the aim has not been satisfied);
- measurable (evidence that the objective has been achieved can be gathered).

Scope concerns where, to whom and to what the project applies – it describes the boundaries and context of the project. Determining an appropriate scope is crucial to the success of any management activity. If the scope is too broad, it is possible that the project will not be completed within the required time. If the scope is too loosely defined, it is possible to stray into areas and topics that are not directly related to the subject and that will not contribute to the project. Authorization will be required for the project aim, objectives, and particularly the scope.

To determine the authority for the project, the following questions may be asked.

- Under whose authority does the project fall?
- To whom does the project manager report?
- Who will ensure the project's implementation?

Context is crucial to planning and implementing an emergency preparedness programme. Before emergency planning and vulnerability assessment are carried out, it is necessary to:

- be familiar with the cultural background of the community;
- determine community attitudes to hazards and emergencies;

— identify local organizations with resources and expertise;
— analyse the political structure of the community and identify those who have power and influence.

The context of emergency preparedness is the "real world" within which the programme must function. If the programme is not adapted to this, it will fail.

A project manager for the emergency preparedness programme should be selected according to the following criteria:

— commitment to the project's success;
— knowledge of the community's culture;
— emergency management knowledge and skills;
— management skills such as team-building, delegating, managing performance, managing others' involvement, communication, negotiation, and conflict resolution;
— problem-solving and decision-making skills;
— project management skills.

Project planning

Project planning is the process of sequencing tasks to achieve the project objectives and to ensure timely project completion and efficient use of resources. It involves determining tasks, assigning responsibilities, developing a timetable, and determining resource allocation and timing.

To determine tasks, the following steps can be taken:

- List the project tasks or steps.
- Determine the time required to complete each task.
- Identify the overall project starting date and project completion date if they have not already been determined.
- List the project tasks, and their starting and completion dates, in the order in which they need to be completed to meet the overall project completion date.

Responsibility for each task or group of tasks should be assigned to competent people. These people should communicate regularly during the performance of their tasks to ensure appropriate coordination. The timetable should take into account all the contributions and work required for the project and should thus be based on the project process and tasks. The timetable will partially determine the resource requirements by indicating the amount of work required, and, therefore, the cost. Resource requirements for the project means "what is needed to get it done?" The following should be listed:

— the expected outputs (some of which will be similar to the objectives);
— the things that need to be done (e.g. meetings, telephone calls, and travel);
— the inputs (resources) in terms of people, materials, time, and money.

Project implementation

The management of project implementation consists of project performance, monitoring, and control; and taking corrective action.

Project monitoring and control is the process of determining progress in accomplishing project objectives. Its purpose is to ensure that the project is implemented successfully and that problems and opportunities are responded to quickly. It also allows a quick return to the project plan if the project strays off schedule.

An effective project monitoring and control system depends on having a clear standard of performance and providing feedback on project performance so that effective action can be taken. Project monitoring and control systems are based on three fundamental steps:

— measuring the progress toward project objectives according to the project timetable;
— determining the cause of deviations in project progress;
— identifying corrective actions through the use of potential problem analysis.

Reference

1. *Project management.* Princeton, NJ, Kepner-Tregoe, 1987.

Annex 2
Hazard description tables

Tables A2.1 to A2.9 on the following pages can provide assistance in describing some hazards.

Table A2.1. **Beaufort scale**[a]

No.	Wind speed km/h	Wind speed knots	Descriptive term	Effects observed On land	Effects observed On sea
0	<1	<1	Calm	Calm; smoke rises vertically	Sea like a mirror
1	1–5	1–3	Light air	Smoke drift indicates wind direction	Ripples are formed but without foam crests
2	6–11	3–6	Light breeze	Leaves rustle; wind vanes move	Small wavelets; crests have a glassy appearance and do not break
3	12–19	6–10	Gentle breeze	Leaves, small twigs in constant motion	Large wavelets; crests begin to break; foam of glassy appearance
4	20–28	11–15	Moderate breeze	Dust, leaves and loose paper raised from ground; small branches move	Small waves, becoming longer; fairly frequent white horses
5	29–38	16–21	Fresh breeze	Small trees in leaf begin to sway	Moderate waves; many white horses formed
6	39–49	21–27	Strong breeze	Larger tree branches in motion; whistling heard in wires	Large waves begin to form; white foam crests everywhere (probably some spray)
7	50–61	27–33	Near gale	Whole trees in motion; difficulty in walking	Sea heaps up; white foam from breaking waves begins to be blown in streaks
8	62–74	33–40	Gale	Twigs and small branches broken off trees; walking impeded	Moderately high waves of greater length; foam is blown in well-marked streaks
9	75–88	41–48	Strong gale	Slight damage to structures; slates blown from roofs	High waves; crests of waves begin to topple, tumble and roll over
10	89–102	48–55	Storm	Trees broken or uprooted; considerable damage to structures	Very high waves with long over-hanging crests; on the whole the surface of the sea takes on a white appearance; the tumbling of the sea becomes heavy and shock-like; visibility affected
11	103–117	56–63	Violent storm	Usually widespread damage	Exceptionally high waves; visibility affected
12	>117	>63	Hurricane	Usually widespread damage	The air is filled with foam and spray; sea completely white with driving spray; visibility seriously affected

[a] Reproduced from reference *1* by permission of the publisher.

Table A2.2. **Hurricane disaster potential scale**[a]

No.	Central pressure (mbar)	Winds (km/h)	Surge (m)	Damage On land	At sea
1	>980	120–150	1.2–1.5	Damage to shrubbery, trees, foliage and poorly anchored mobile homes. Some damage to signs.	Some low-lying coastal roads flooded. Limited damage to piers and exposed small craft.
2	965–979	151–175	1.6–2.4	Trees stripped of foliage and some of them broken down. Exposed mobile homes suffer major damage. Poorly constructed signs are severely damaged. Some roofing material ripped off; windows and doors might be affected.	Coastal roads and escape routes flooded 2–4 hours before hurricane centre arrives. Piers suffer extensive damage and small unprotected craft are torn loose. Some evacuation of coastal areas is necessary.
3	945–964	175–210	2.5–3.6	Foliage stripped from trees and many blown down. Great damage to roofing material, doors and windows. Some small buildings are structurally damaged.	Serious coastal flooding and some coastal buildings may be damaged. Battering of waves might affect large buildings, but not severely. Coastal escape routes cut off 3–5 hours before hurricane centre arrives. Flat terrain 1.5 m or less above sea level is flooded as far inland as 13 km. Evacuation of coastal residents for several blocks inland may be necessary.
4	920–944	211–250	3.7–5.5	Shrubs, trees and signs are all blown down. Extensive damage to roofing materials, doors and windows. Many roofs on smaller buildings may be ripped off. Mobile homes destroyed.	Flat land up to 3 m above sea level might be flooded to 10 km inland. Extensive damage to the lower floors of buildings near the coast. Escape routes cut 3–5 hours before hurricane centre passes. Beaches suffer major erosion, and evacuation of homes within 500 m of coast may be necessary.
5	<920	>250	>5.5	Increase on the extensive damage of the previous level. Glass in windows shattered and many structures blown over.	Lower floors of structures within 500 m of coast extensively damaged. Escape routes cut off 3–5 hours before hurricane centre arrives. Evacuation of low lying areas within 8–16 km of coast may be necessary.

[a] Reproduced from reference 2 by permission of the publisher and the author.

Table A2.3. **Frequency of tropical storms**[a]

Basin and stage	Jan.	Feb.	Mar.	Apr.	May	June	July	Aug.	Sep.	Oct.	Nov.	Dec.	Annual
North Atlantic													
Tropical storms	*	*	*	*	0.1	0.4	0.3	1.0	1.5	1.2	0.4	*	4.2
Hurricanes	*	*	*	*	*	0.3	0.4	1.5	2.7	1.3	0.3	*	5.2
Tropical storms and hurricanes	*	*	*	*	0.2	0.7	0.8	2.5	4.3	2.5	0.7	0.1	9.4
Eastern north Pacific													
Tropical storms	*	*	*	*	*	1.5	2.8	2.3	2.3	1.2	0.3	*	9.3
Hurricanes	*	*	*	*	0.3	0.6	0.9	2.0	1.8	1.0	*	*	5.8
Tropical storms and hurricanes	*	*	*	*	0.3	2.0	3.6	4.5	4.1	2.2	0.3	*	15.2
Western north Pacific													
Tropical storms	0.2	0.3	0.3	0.2	0.4	0.5	1.2	1.8	1.5	1.0	0.8	0.6	7.5
Typhoons	0.3	0.2	0.2	0.7	0.9	1.2	2.7	4.0	4.1	3.3	2.1	0.7	17.8
Tropical storms and typhoons	0.4	0.4	0.5	0.9	1.3	1.8	3.9	5.8	5.6	4.3	2.9	1.3	25.3
Southwest Pacific and Australian area													
Tropical storms	2.7	2.8	2.4	1.3	0.3	0.2	*	*	*	0.1	0.4	1.5	10.9
Typhoons/cyclones	0.7	1.1	1.3	0.3	*	*	0.1	0.1	*	*	0.3	0.5	3.8
Tropical storms and typhoons/cyclones	3.4	4.1	3.7	1.7	0.3	0.2	0.1	0.1	*	0.1	0.7	2.0	14.8
Southwest Indian Ocean													
Tropical storms	2.0	2.2	1.7	0.6	0.2	*	*	*	*	0.3	0.3	0.8	7.4
Cyclones	1.3	1.1	0.8	0.4	*	*	*	*	*	*	*	0.5	3.8
Tropical storms and cyclones	3.2	3.3	2.5	1.1	0.2	*	*	*	*	0.3	0.4	1.4	11.2
North Indian Ocean													
Tropical storms	0.1	*	*	0.1	0.3	0.5	0.5	0.4	0.4	0.6	0.5	0.3	3.5
Cyclones[b]	*	*	*	0.1	0.5	0.2	0.1	*	0.1	0.4	0.6	0.2	2.2
Tropical storms and cyclones[b]	0.1	*	0.1	0.3	0.7	0.7	0.6	0.4	0.5	1.0	1.1	0.5	5.7

[a] Reproduced from reference 1 by permission of the publisher.
[b] Winds >89 km/h (Beaufort 10).
* Less than 0.05.
Note: Monthly values cannot be combined because single storms overlapping two months were counted once in each month and once annually.

Table A2.4. **Modified Mercalli scale**[a]

No.	Descriptive term	Description[b]	Acceleration $(cm\,s^{-2})$
I	Imperceptible	Not felt. Marginal and long-period effects of large earthquakes.	<1
II	Very slight	Felt by persons at rest, on upper floor, or favourably placed.	1–2
III	Slight	Felt indoors. Hanging objects swing. Vibration like passing of light trucks. Duration estimated. May not be recognised as an earthquake.	2–5
IV	Moderate	Hanging objects swing. Vibration like passing of heavy trucks or sensation of a jolt like a heavy ball striking the walls. Standing motor cars rock. Windows, dishes, doors rattle. Glasses clink, crockery clashes. In upper range of IV, wooden walls and frames creak.	5–10
V	Rather strong	Felt outdoors; direction estimated. Sleepers waken. Liquids disturbed, some spilled. Small unstable objects displaced or upset. Doors swing, close, open. Shutters, pictures move. Pendulum clocks stop, start, change rate.	10–20
VI	Strong	Felt by all. Many frightened and run outdoors. People walk unsteadily. Dishes, glassware broken. Knick-knacks, books, off shelves. Pictures off walls. Furniture overturned or moved. Weak plaster, masonry D cracked. Small bells ring. Trees shaken.	20–50
VII	Very strong	Difficult to stand. Noticed by motor car drivers. Hanging objects quiver. Furniture broken. Damage to masonry D, including cracks. Weak chimneys broken at roof line. Fall of plaster, loose bricks, stones, tiles, cornices. Some cracks in masonry C. Waves on ponds: water turbid with mud. Small slides and caving in along sand or gravel banks. Large bells ring. Concrete irrigation ditches damaged.	50–100
VIII	Destructive	Steering of motor cars affected. Damage to masonry C: partial collapse. Some damage to masonry B, none to masonry A. Fall of stucco, some masonry walls. Twisting, fall of chimneys, factory stacks, monuments, towers, elevated tanks. Frame houses move on foundations if not bolted down; loose panel walls thrown out. Decayed piling broken off. Branches broken from trees. Changes in flow or temperature of springs and wells. Cracks in wet ground, on steep slopes.	100–200
IX	Devastating	General panic. Masonry D destroyed; masonry C heavily damaged, sometimes with complete collapse; masonry B seriously damaged. Frame structures, if not bolted, shifted off foundations. Frames cracked. Serious damage to reservoirs. Underground pipes broken. Conspicuous cracks in ground. In alluviated areas sand and mud ejected, earthquake fountains, sand craters.	200–500
X	Annihilating	Most masonry and frame structures destroyed with their foundations. Some well-built wooden structures and bridges destroyed. Serious damage to dams, dykes, and embankments. Large landslides. Water thrown on banks of canals, rivers, lakes, etc. Sand and mud shifted horizontally on beaches and flat land. Rails bent slightly.	500–1000

Table A2.4 (continued)

No.	Descriptive term	Description	Acceleration (cm s^{-2})
XI	Disaster	Rails bent greatly. Underground pipelines completely out of service.	1000–2000
XII	Major Disaster	Damage nearly total. Large rockmasses displaced. Line of sight and level distorted. Objects thrown into the air.	>2000

[a] Reproduced from reference 1 by permission of the publisher.
[b] Masonry A: Good workmanship, mortar and design; reinforced, especially laterally, and bound together using steel, concrete, etc.; designed to resist lateral forces.
Masonry B: Good workmanship and mortar; reinforced, but not designed in detail to resist lateral forces.
Masonry C: Ordinary workmanship and mortar; no extreme weaknesses like failing to tie in at corners, but neither reinforced nor designed against horizontal forces.
Masonry D: Weak materials, such as adobe; poor mortar; low standards of workmanship; weak horizontally.

Table A2.5. **Landslide damage intensity scale**[a]

Grade	Description of damage	
0	None	Building is intact.
1	Negligible	Hairline cracks in walls or structural members: no distortion of structure or detachment of external architectural details.
2	Light	Building continues to be habitable; repair not urgent. Settlement of foundations, distortion of structure and inclination of walls are not sufficient to compromise overall stability.
3	Moderate	Walls out of perpendicular by 1–2°, or substantial cracking has occurred to structural members, or foundations have settled during differential subsidence of at least 15 cm: building requires evacuation and rapid attention to ensure its continued life.
4	Serious	Walls out of perpendicular by several degrees; open cracks in walls; fracture of structural members; fragmentation of masonry; differential settlement of at least 25 cm compromises foundations; floors may be inclined by 1–2°, or ruined by soil heave; internal partition walls will need to be replaced; door and window frames too distorted to use; occupants must be evacuated and major repairs carried out.
5	Very serious	Walls out of plumb by 5–6°; structure grossly distorted and differential settlement will have seriously cracked floors and walls or caused major rotation or slewing of the building (wooden buildings may have detached completely from their foundations). Partition walls and brick infill will have at least partly collapsed: roof may have partially collapsed; outhouses, porches and patios may have been damaged more seriously than the principal structure itself. Occupants will need to be rehoused on a long-term basis, and rehabilitation of the building will probably not be feasible.
6	Partial collapse	Requires immediate evacuation of the occupants and cordoning off the site to prevent accidents from falling masonry.
7	Total collapse	Requires clearance of the site.

[a] Reproduced from reference 2 by permission of the publisher and the author.

Table A2.6. **Example of a damage probability matrix for landslides**[a]
(Failure probability for a slope of low stability, summer conditions, earthquake shaking of various intensities)

Degree of slope failure	Probability of slope failure in earthquake ground-shaking intensity				
	VI	VII	VIII	IX	X
Light	40%	25%	15%	10%	5%
Moderate	30%	30%	35%	30%	20%
Heavy	25%	35%	40%	40%	35%
Severe	5%	10%	10%	15%	30%
Catastrophic	0%	0%	0%	5%	10%

[a] Reproduced from reference 3 by permission of the publisher.

Table A2.7. **Tsunami intensity scale**[a]

Intensity	Run-up height (m)	Descriptive term	Description
I	0.5	Very light	Waves so weak as to be perceptible only on tide gauge records.
II	1	Light	Waves noticed by those living along the shore and familiar with the sea. On very flat shores generally noticed.
III	1	Rather strong	Generally noticed. Flooding of gently sloping coasts. Light sailing vessels carried away on shore. Slight damage to light structures situated near coast. In estuaries reversal of river flow for some distance upstream.
IV	4	Strong	Flooding of the shore to some depth. Light scouring on man-made ground. Embankments and dykes damaged. Light structures near the coast damaged. Solid structures on the coast slightly damaged. Big sailing vessels and small ships drifted inland or carried out to sea. Coasts littered with floating debris.
V	8	Very strong	General flooding of the shore to some depth. Quay walls and solid structures near the sea damaged. Light structures destroyed. Severe scouring of cultivated land and littering of the coast with floating items and sea animals. With the exception of big ships all other types of vessels carried inland or out to sea. Big bores in estuary rivers. Harbour works damaged. People drowned, waves accompanied by strong roar.
VI	16	Disastrous	Partial or complete destruction of man-made structures for some distance from the shore. Flooding of coasts to great depths. Big ships severely damaged. Trees uprooted or broken by the waves. Many casualties.

[a] Reproduced from reference 1 by permission of the publisher.

Table A2.8. **Volcanic eruption scales**[a]

Volcanic explosivity index (VEI)	Volcanic intensity	Tsuya scale	Eruption rate (kg/s)	Volume of ejecta (m^3)	Eruption column height (km)	Thermal power output (log kW)	Duration (hours of continuous blast)
0	V	I	10^2–10^3	$<10^4$	0.8–1.5	5–6	<1
1	VI	II–III	10^3–10^4	10^4–10^6	1.5–2.8	6–7	<1
2	VII	IV	10^4–10^5	10^6–10^7	2.8–5.5	7–8	1–6
3	VIII	V	10^5–10^6	10^7–10^8	5.5–10.5	8–9	1–12
4	IX	VI	10^6–10^7	10^8–10^9	10.5–17.0	9–10	1–>12
5	X	VII	10^7–10^8	10^9–10^{10}	17.0–28.0	10–11	6–>12
6	XI	VIII	10^8–10^9	10^{10}–10^{11}	28.0–47.0	11–12	>12
7	XII	IX	$>10^9$	10^{11}–10^{12}	>47.0	>12	>12
8	—	—	—	$>10^{12}$	—	—	>12

[a] Reproduced from reference 2 by permission of the publisher and the author.

Table A2.9. **Dangerous goods classes**[a]

Class 1 — Explosives	—	—
Class 2 — Gases: compressed, liquefied or dissolved under pressure	Class 2.1	Flammable gases
	Class 2.2	Non-flammable non-toxic gases
	Class 2.3	Toxic gases
Class 3 — Flammable liquids	Class 3.1	Liquids with a flashpoint below −18°C (closed cup test)
	Class 3.2	Liquids with a flashpoint of −18°C up to but not including 23°C (closed cup test)
	Class 3.3	Liquids with a flashpoint of 23°C or more, up to and including 61°C (closed cup test)
Class 4 — Flammable solids	Class 4.1	Flammable solids
	Class 4.2	Substances liable to spontaneous combustion
	Class 4.3	Substances which emit flammable gases on contact with water
Class 5 — Oxidizing substances (agents) and organic peroxides	Class 5.1	Oxidizing agents
	Class 5.2	Organic peroxides
Class 6 — Toxic and infectious substances	Class 6.1	Toxic substances
	Class 6.2	Infectious substances
Class 7 — Radioactive substances	—	—
Class 8 — Corrosives	—	—
Class 9 — Miscellaneous dangerous substances and articles	—	—

[a] Reproduced and updated from reference 4 by permission of the publisher.

References

1. *Technical insurance references.* Münchener Ruckversicherungs-Gesellschaft [Munich Reinsurance], Munich, 1984.

2. Alexander DE. *Natural disasters.* London, University College London Press, 1993.

3. Coburn AW et al. *Vulnerability and risk assessment.* Geneva, Office of the United Nations Disaster Relief Coordinator and United Nations Development Programme, 1991.

4. *International maritime dangerous goods code.* Geneva, International Maritime Organization, 1986.

Annex 3
Emergency preparedness checklists

The checklists in this annex can be used for developing or evaluating emergency preparedness programmes. Some parts of the checklists would also be of value during response and recovery operations.

Policy

- Have all emergency management parts of relevant legislation been located, and have the implications of this legislation been considered in community emergency preparedness?
- Have any inconsistencies in the legislation been reported to central government?
- Is there power for the following actions during emergencies:
  — commandeering of resources?
  — evacuation of people at risk?
  — centralized coordination of emergency work at the national, provincial, and community levels?

Vulnerability assessment

- Is a vulnerability assessment available for emergency preparedness, as well as for emergency response and recovery work?
- Are there procedures for reviewing vulnerability assessment in the light of:
  — community change?
  — vulnerability change?
  — hazards change?
  — capacity/capability change?

Planning

- Have private organizations and NGOs been involved in the planning process?
- Has assistance or guidance in developing emergency plans been provided to government, private organizations, and NGOs?
- Are there emergency plans that are related to the community emergency plan?
- If such plans exist, what are the implications for your plans?
- Has contact been made with people in other organizations or jurisdictional areas who may be able to assist the community?
- Has the plan been approved by the chief executive of the community administration?

- Has the plan been endorsed by all relevant organizations?
- Has a person or organization been assigned responsibility for developing the community emergency plan?
- Who is responsible for keeping the emergency plan up to date and how often is it to be formally reviewed?
- Do people who hold existing plans receive amendments?
- Is a distribution list of the plan maintained?
- Have the community emergency management structure and organizational responsibilities been described?
- Who is responsible for the overall management?
- Who is responsible for the operations of particular organizations?
- Who is responsible for coordinating particular tasks?
- Are all the necessary tasks assigned to organizations and personnel?
- Are the responsibilities of all organizations described?
- Does the plan contain a summary of the vulnerability assessment?
- Has the relationship between different levels of planning been described?
- Have mutual aid and twinning agreements with adjacent communities been made?
- Is the plan consistent with related plans?
- Does the plan make reference to the legislation that establishes the legal basis for planning and carrying out emergency measures?

Training and education

- Who is responsible for the various training and education requirements of emergency workers and the public?
- Has a training needs analysis of emergency workers been performed?
- Have a number of different public education strategies been implemented?
- How quickly are new personnel in organizations made capable of working in emergency management?
- Is institutional memory being preserved? For example, do people have to "reinvent the wheel" or are past, practical lessons learned, documented, and passed on?
- Do the capabilities and capacities of organizations improve over time during the implementation of preparedness strategies?

Monitoring and evaluation

- Is there a procedure for reviewing emergency preparedness on a regular or as-required basis? How is it done and who is responsible?
- How often is the community plan to be exercised? Who is responsible?
- How are the lessons learned from exercises to be incorporated into plans?
- Are multi-organizational exercises run, as well as single-organizational exercises?

Communications

- What forms of communication are available?
- Are there backups?
- Who is responsible for communications maintenance and planning?

- Do people know the relevant radio frequencies and contact numbers?
- Are there contact lists (containing names, telephone numbers, etc.) for all emergency management organizations?
- Do the communications systems allow communication between all relevant organizations?

Search and rescue

- What rescue tasks may need to be performed?
- Who is responsible, who coordinates?
- Are there procedures for detecting and marking danger areas?
- How are search and rescue activities integrated with other emergency functions, in particular health?

Health and medical

- Have the ambulance and hospital services planned and been trained for the handling of mass casualties?
- Are they aware of each other's arrangements?
- Are there emergency field medical teams?
- Who manages these on-site?
- Are there arrangements for counselling the public and emergency workers? Who is responsible for providing this service and who pays for it?

Social welfare

- Are the arrangements for feeding and accommodating people linked to the registration and enquiry system and the evacuation procedures?
- Is there any arrangement for expediting the assessment of damage to private and public property and payment for losses?
- Do the insurance companies have any cooperative arrangements among themselves?
- Where, when, and how do people have access to insurance companies?
- What is insurance company policy on makeshift repairs or repairs to minimize damage?
- Is there access to legal advisers during emergency response and recovery operations?
- Is there a system for providing legal advice to emergency-affected persons?

Transport and lifelines

- Who is responsible for each lifeline?
- What are the priorities for repairing damaged lifelines?
- How long should it take to repair each lifeline from the predicted levels of damage?
- How are alternative lifelines to be arranged if required?

Police and investigation

- Are there procedures to ensure that resources are reserved from the emergency response work to enforce law and order?

Alerting

- Who is responsible for receiving warnings from outside the community?
- Is there a clear system that ensures that all relevant organizations and personnel are alerted?
- Does this system:
  — assign responsibility for initiating an alert?
  — provide for a "cascade" method of alerting, whereby those alerted are responsible for further alerting where appropriate?
  — describe the first actions required by those alerted?
  — provide for the cancellation of an alert and the stand-down of organizations and personnel?

Command, control and coordination

- Is there a threat to the existence or continuity of government?
- Who is responsible for planning for continuity of government?
- Have all senior management personnel and elected officials been allocated a task?
- To whom do management personnel or officials turn for information?
- Are there procedures for ensuring the safety of government and administrative records (paper and computerized)?
- Have lines of succession been determined to ensure continuity of leadership?
- Have alternative sites for government organizations been identified?
- Have locations for emergency coordination centres been designated and promulgated?
- Are there alternative centres?
- Are they remote from areas likely to be damaged?
- Do they have adequate communications, feeding, sleeping, and sanitation facilities?
- Do they have backup power?
- Is the availability of backup communications equipment known?
- Is there an adequate water supply?
- Is there a designated centre manager and alternative and relieving managers?
- Do the centres have trained staff?
- Are there procedures for developing staff rosters?
- Are there procedures for activating and operating the centres?
- Is there adequate administrative support for the centres?
- Are functions of the centres succinctly described?
- Is there a procedure method for collecting, verifying, analysing, and disseminating information?
- Is there a procedure for recording events, requests for assistance, decisions, and allocating resources?
- Are there internal security arrangements for the centres?
- Has responsibility for day-to-day maintenance of the centres been assigned?
- Are there procedures within and between organizations for the briefing of personnel on an impending or actual emergency?

- Are there procedures for conducting single and multi-organizational debriefings following an emergency or alert?

Information management
- Are maps of the community (topographic, demographic, hazard, and vulnerability) available?
- Is a public information centre designated as the official point of contact by public and the media during an emergency?
- Are there provisions for releasing information to the public, including appropriate protective actions and devised responses?
- Have agreements been reached with the media for disseminating public information and emergency warnings?
- Are contact details for all media outlets (radio, television, and newspapers) available?
- Who is responsible for providing information to the media?
- Who is responsible for authorizing information?
- Who is responsible for emergency assessment and to whom do they report? How is the information recorded and who relays the information to those concerned?
- Who is responsible for issuing public statements about emergencies?
- Do they have public credibility and adequate liaison with other organizations who may also issue warnings?
- Who is responsible for providing warnings for each likely type of emergency?
- To whom is the warning supplied?
- At which warning level is response action initiated?
- What is the purpose of the warnings and what action is required of the public?
- Who will inform the public when the danger has passed?
- Is there a point of contact for members of the public wanting specific information, and is this point of contact publicly known?
- Is there a referral service for directing people to the appropriate sources of information?
- Is there a registration and enquiry system for recording the whereabouts of displaced, injured, or dead persons?
- Is there a system for providing this information to bona fide inquirers?
- Does the community know how to contact the registration and inquiry system?
- Is there a facility for multilingual message broadcasting and an interpreter service for incoming calls?
- Are there plans for establishing public information centres?
- Is the community aware of the existence of these centres?

Resource management
- Who coordinates resources within each organization?
- Who is responsible for supplying resources beyond the normal capabilities of each organization? Who records the use and cost of resources?
- Have arrangements been made with national or provincial military organizations for assistance in times of emergency?

- Is there agreed access to emergency funds?
- Who records the expenditure for future acquittal/repayment?
- What are the limits of expenditure for personnel?
- What tasks can be safely performed by unskilled volunteers?
- Who coordinates this work?
- Is it likely that some organizations will begin public appeals for donations to emergency-affected persons?
- How can these appeals be coordinated?
- How is equitable disbursement of appeal money to be ensured?
- Who coordinates the requests for assistance for the community?
- What sort of assistance is likely to be required?
- Where is this assistance likely to come from?
- Is there an expected form that the request should take?
- Is the following information available to help outside assistance:
  — lists of organizations working in the country, with information on their competence and capacity to be involved in emergency response and recovery activities?
  — lists of essential response and recovery items not available in the community that would need to be obtained abroad, with available information on potential international sources?
  — information on customs and taxation regulations covering the importation and transit of response and recovery (and other) items?
- Is the following information available:
  — lists of essential response and recovery items, with specifications and average costs?
  — lists of local manufacturers and regional manufacturers or suppliers of response and recovery items, with information on quality, capacity and capability, delivery times, and reliability?
  — information on essential response and recovery resources that will allow a rapid response, e.g. water supply systems, sanitation systems, health networks, alternative shelter sites and materials, ports and transport networks, warehouses, and communications systems?

Evacuation

- Does any person or organization have the authority to evacuate people who are threatened?
- Are there designated locations to which evacuees should travel?
- How many people may need to be evacuated?
- In what circumstances should they be evacuated?
- Who will tell people that it is safe to return? What will trigger this?
- Are staging areas and pick-up points identified for evacuation?
- Are evacuees to be provided with information on where they are going and how they will be cared for?
- Is there security for evacuated areas?
- How are prisoners to be evacuated?
- How are the cultural and religious requirements of evacuees to be catered for?
- Who is responsible for traffic control during evacuation?
- How are evacuees to be registered?

Response and recovery operations

- Has a community emergency committee been set up?
- Have response teams been organized?
- Is anything being done for isolated families?
- Have arrangements been made to pick up the injured and take them to the health centre or hospital?
- Have people been evacuated from dangerous buildings?
- Have steps been taken to resolve the most urgent problems for the survival of the victims, including water, food, and shelter?
- Has a place been assigned for the dead to be kept while awaiting burial?
- Are steps being taken to identify the dead?
- Has an information centre been established?
- Have communications been established with the central (regional, national) government?
- Has there been a needs assessment to consider the number of people needing assistance, the type of assistance required, and the resources locally available?
- Are steps being taken to reunite families?
- Have safety instructions been issued?
- Are steps being taken to circulate information on:
  — the consequences of the emergency?
  — the dangers that exist?
  — facts that may reassure people?
- Are communications being maintained with the central government?
- Is information on requirements being coordinated?
- Are local volunteer workers being coordinated?
- Are volunteer workers from outside being coordinated?
- Is inappropriate aid being successfully prevented and avoided?
- Are response and recovery supplies being fairly distributed?
- Is contact being maintained with all family groupings?
- Have families who are living in buildings that are damaged but not dangerous been reassured?
- Has an appropriate site been chosen for temporary shelters?
- In setting up shelters for emergency victims, have family and neighbourhood relationships and socioeconomic and cultural needs been taken into account?
- Have the victims been organized in family groupings?
- Have the essential problems been dealt with:
  — water supply?
  — the provision of clothing, footwear, and blankets?
  — food supply?
  — facilities for preparing hot meals?
  — the installation of latrines?
  — facilities for washing clothes and pots and pans?
  — collection and disposal of waste?
- Have short meetings been arranged in the community to discuss the various problems and find solutions to them?

- Have steps been taken to encourage solidarity, mutual assistance, and constructive efforts among the people?
- Have school activities started up again?
- Have initiatives been taken for community action by children?
- Have steps been take to combat false rumours?
- Have measures been adopted to ensure that there is no favouritism in the distribution of response and recovery supplies?
- Is care being taken to make certain that volunteer workers from outside do not take the place of local people but help them to take the situation in hand?
- Have the victims been encouraged and helped to resume their activities?
- Have initiatives been taken to facilitate economic recovery, putting local resources to good use?
- Have steps been taken to ensure that people participate in drawing up plans of recovery and development and that those plans are in line with needs and the local culture?
- Are arrangements in force to avoid:
  — delays?
  — crippling disputes?
  — favouritism?
  — speculation?
  — dishonesty?
  — violence?

References

1. *Australian emergency manual: community emergency planning guide*, 2nd ed. Canberra, Natural Disasters Organisation, 1992.

2. *A guide for the review of state and local emergency operations plans.* Washington, DC, Federal Emergency Management Agency, 1992 (CPG 1–8A).

3. *Capability assessment and standards for state and local government (interim guidance).* Washington, DC, Federal Emergency Management Agency, 1983 (CPG 1–102).

4. International Civil Defence Organisation. The international status of civil defence and the ICDO. *International civil defence journal*, 1993, 6(3):44–46.

5. Koob PC. *Planning process II.* Hobart, University of Tasmania, 1993.

Annex 4
Personal protection in different types of emergencies

Introduction

In addition to considering action by rescuers, thought must be given to personal protection measures in different types of emergencies. While such measures may not directly contribute to saving casualties, they help to reduce their number. By taking precautions, the individual assists the collective effort to reduce the effects of an emergency. The types of emergency considered here are:

— floods;
— storms, hurricanes, and tornadoes;
— earthquakes;
— clouds of toxic fumes.

A number of measures must be observed by *all* persons in *all* types of emergency:

- Do not use the telephone, except to call for help, so as to leave telephone lines free for the organization of response.
- Listen to the messages broadcast by radio and the various media so as to be informed of development.
- Carry out the official instructions given over the radio or by loudspeaker.
- Keep a family emergency kit ready.

In all the different types of emergency, it is better:

— to be prepared than to get hurt;
— to get information so as to get organized;
— to wait rather than act too hastily.

Floods

What to do beforehand

While town planning is a government responsibility, individuals should find out about risks in the area where they live. For example, people who live in areas downstream from a dam should know the special signals (such as foghorns) used when a dam threatens to break. Small floods can be foreseen by watching the water level after heavy rains and regularly listening to the weather forecasts.

Forecasting of floods or tidal waves is very difficult, but hurricanes and cyclones often occur at the same time of year, when particular vigilance must be exercised. They are often announced several hours or days before they arrive.

During a flood
- Turn off the electricity to reduce the risk of electrocution.
- Protect people and property:
  — as soon as the flood begins, take any vulnerable people (children, the old, the sick, and the disabled) to an upper floor;
  — whenever possible, move personal belongings upstairs or go to raised shelters provided for use in floods.
- Beware of water contamination — if the taste, colour, or smell of the water is suspicious, it is vital to use some means of purification.
- Evacuate danger zones as ordered by the local authorities — it is essential to comply strictly with the evacuation advice given. Authorities will recommend that families take with them the emergency supplies they have prepared.

After a flood
When a flood is over, it is important that people do not return home until told to do so by the local authorities, who will have ensured that buildings have not been undermined by water. From then on it is essential to:

— wait until the water is declared safe before drinking any that is untreated;
— clean and disinfect any room that has been flooded;
— sterilize or wash with boiling water all dishes and kitchen utensils;
— get rid of any food that has been in or near the water, including canned foods and any food kept in refrigerators and freezers;
— get rid of all consumables (drinks, medicines, cosmetics, etc.).

Storms, hurricanes and tornadoes

What to do beforehand
Above all, it is vital that people find out about the kinds of storm liable to strike their region so that they can take optimum preventive measures, and:

— choose a shelter in advance, before the emergency occurs — a cellar, a basement, or an alcove may be perfectly suitable;
— minimize the effects of the storm — fell dead trees, prune tree branches, regularly check the state of roofs, the state of the ground, and the drainage around houses;
— take measures against flooding;
— prepare a family emergency kit.

During an emergency
- Listen to the information and advice provided by the authorities.
- Do not go out in a car or a boat once the storm has been announced.
- Evacuate houses if the authorities request this, taking the family emergency package.
- If possible, tie down any object liable to be blown away by the wind; if there is time, nail planks to the doors and shutters, open the windows and doors slightly on the side opposite to the direction from which the wind is coming so as to reduce wind pressure on the house.

- If caught outside in a storm, take refuge as quickly as possible in a shelter; if there is no shelter, lie down flat in a ditch.
- In a thunderstorm keep away from doors, windows, and electrical conductors, unplug electrical appliances and television aerials. Do not use any electrical appliances or the telephone.
- Anyone who is outside should:
  — look for shelter in a building (never under a tree);
  — if out in a boat, get back to the shore;
  — keep away from fences and electric cables;
  — kneel down rather than remain standing.

After an emergency
After the storm has subsided:

— follow the instructions given by the authorities;
— stay indoors and do not go to the stricken areas;
— give the alert as quickly as possible;
— give first aid to the injured;
— make sure the water is safe to drink and check the contents of refrigerators and freezers;
— check the exterior of dwellings and call for assistance if there is a risk of falling objects (tiles, guttering, etc.).

Earthquakes

What to do beforehand
The movement of the ground in an earthquake is rarely the direct cause of injuries; most are caused by falling objects or collapsing buildings. Many earthquakes are followed (several hours or even days later) by further tremors, usually of progressively decreasing intensity. To reduce the destructive effects of earthquakes a number of precautions are essential for people living in risk areas:

- Build in accordance with urban planning regulations for risk areas.
- Ensure that all electrical and gas appliances in houses, together with all pipes connected to them, are firmly fixed.
- Avoid storing heavy objects and materials in high positions.
- Hold family evacuation drills and ensure that the whole family knows what to do in case of an earthquake.
- Prepare a family emergency kit.

During an earthquake
- Keep calm, do not panic.
- People who are indoors should stay there but move to the central part of the building.
- Keep away from the stairs, which might collapse suddenly.
- People who are outside should stay there, keeping away from buildings to avoid collapsing walls and away from electric cables.
- Anyone in a vehicle should park it, keeping away from bridges and buildings.

After an earthquake
- Obey the authorities' instructions.
- Do not go back into damaged buildings since tremors may start again at any moment.
- Give first aid to the injured and alert the emergency services in case of fire, burst pipes, etc.
- Do not go simply to look at the stricken areas: this will hamper rescue work.
- Keep emergency packages and a radio near at hand.
- Make sure that water is safe to drink and food stored at home is fit to eat (in case of electricity cuts affecting refrigerators and freezers).

Clouds of toxic fumes

What to do beforehand
People in a risk area should:

— find out about evacuation plans and facilities;
— familiarize themselves with the alarm signals used in case of emergency;
— equip doors and windows with the tightest possible fastenings;
— prepare family emergency kits.

During an emergency
- Do not use the telephone; leave lines free for rescue services.
- Listen to the messages given by radio and other media.
- Carry out the instructions transmitted by radio or loudspeaker.
- Close doors and windows.
- Stop up air intakes.
- Seal any cracks or gaps around windows and doors with adhesive tape.
- Organize a reserve of water (by filling wash basins, baths, etc.).
- Turn off ventilators and air conditioners.

After an emergency
- Comply with the authorities' instructions and do not go out until there is no longer any risk.
- Carry out necessary decontamination measures.